A Way of Thinking

A Primer on the Art of Being a Doctor

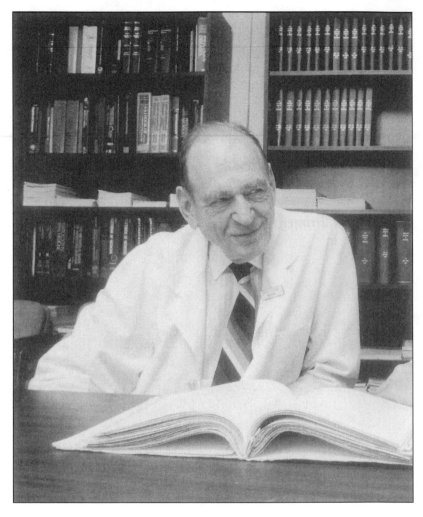

Eugene A. Stead, Jr.

A Way of Thinking

A Primer on the Art of Being a Doctor

Essays by
Eugene A. Stead, Jr., M.D.

Edited by
Barton F. Haynes, M.D.

Carolina Academic Press
Durham, North Carolina

ISBN 0-89089-753-0
LCCN 95-68700

Grateful acknowledgment is made to the following publishers, editors, or authors for permission to reproduce previously published work: Francis A. Countway Library of Medicine, Harvard Medical School, North Carolina Medical Journal, Williams & Wilkins Press, Carolina Academic Press, Decker Periodicals, Drs. Earl Metz and Fred Schoonmaker, American Medical Association, Archives of Internal Medicine, *The Pharos,* Alpha Omega Alpha Honor Medical Society, Duke University Medical Library Trent Collection, The Association of American Physicians, Drs. Eugene A. Stead, Jr., Galen Wagner, and Marvin Rozear, Ms. Bess Cebe, Rockefeller University Press, and *Resident and Staff Physician* for material that appeared in *Medical Times.*

Carolina Academic Press
700 Kent Street
Durham, North Carolina 27701
Telephone (919) 489-7486
Fax (919) 493-5668

Printed in the United States of America

Dedication ⌒

*T*he future of medicine belongs to those who understand not only the principles of molecular medicine, but also the principles of human behavior. This book is dedicated to all health care providers who, in spite of bureaucratic systems, prejudice, and financial disincentives to spend time with patients, continue to care for their patients as human beings with poorly functioning bodies, rather than seeing patients as depersonalized "cases" of disease.

Contents ⌒

Acknowledgments

I am grateful to a number of individuals for their assistance with this book. James Gifford, historian of Duke Medical Center, spent time with me discussing Duke University in the years between 1940 and 1970 and gave me access to many of the photographs I have reprinted. Bess Cebe, Dr. Stead's long-time secretary, unearthed unpublished manuscripts from the Stead files and made helpful comments on this manuscript. Galen Wagner, Irving Holley and Marvin Rozear offered insight into Dr. Stead's way of thinking as well as suggestions about the manuscript. Reynolds Price graciously commented on the book and introduced me to the ways of publishing houses. Jan McCallum, Evelyn Stead and Penny Hodgson provided editorial assistance, and Kim McClammy and Joyce Lowery typed the manuscript and all of Dr. Stead's interviews. My wife, Caroline, and my three children, Charlotte, Ben and Laura, were loving and patient with me during time spent on this project. Finally, I am grateful to Dr. Stead, for his sharing his unpublished material, for allowing me to try to understand his approach to medicine, for his patience with interviews, and for his mentorship.

Barton F. Haynes, M.D.
February, 1995

Introduction ⌒

T his is a book about what it means to be a doctor, how doctors should be educated, and how doctors should strive to continue to educate themselves day by day throughout their careers. The book is also about an extraordinary clinician, teacher, administrator, philosopher and visionary, Eugene A. Stead, Jr., and reflects on how he saw the world of medicine and society in general during his long and productive career at Harvard, Emory, and Duke University Schools of Medicine. Most important, this book is about a way of thinking about medical and societal issues that is unique to Eugene Stead. Therefore, it is important to understand just who Eugene Stead is in order to appreciate the wisdom his words have for us today in the rapidly-changing world of health care reform in the United States.

Born in Atlanta, Georgia in 1908, Eugene Stead was one of five children. His parents were of modest means, yet provided well for the family. Eugene Stead's parents taught the Stead children lessons of honesty and the importance of clear communication between people—lessons that Eugene learned and that formed the foundations for his approach as a physician to science, patients and society. Educated at Emory University undergraduate and medical schools in Atlanta from 1928–1932, Stead benefitted from inspiring mentors such as J. Edgar Paullin, the Stead family physician and staff internist on the faculty of Grady Hospital and Emory Medical School. From Emory, Stead went to Boston for a medical internship at the Peter Bent Brigham

Hospital and an eight month stint in the physiology laboratory. This was followed by a surgical internship at the Brigham and a medicine residency at the Cincinnati General Hospital. From 1937 to 1939, he was the chief resident at the Thorndike Unit at the Boston City Hospital, where he began his research career under a dynamic chief named Soma Weiss. There Stead began his pioneering work on the human circulatory system that culminated in 1944 with J.V. Warren at Emory University in the discovery of the pathophysiology of congestive heart failure. In 1939, Stead gained faculty status at the Harvard Medical School and went with Soma Weiss to the Peter Bent Brigham Hospital. Stead was heavily influenced in Boston by remarkable teachers and clinicians such as Soma Weiss, William Castle, George Minot, Sam Levine, Charles Janeway, John Romano, and Maxwell Finland. In 1942, at the age of 33, Stead went to Emory as Professor and Chairman of Medicine, and after 4½ years, was recruited in 1947 by Wilburt C. Davison, the Dean of the School of Medicine at Duke, to come to Duke as Chairman of Medicine. Stead was Chairman of Medicine at Duke for twenty years, and was succeeded by James B. Wyngaarden in 1967. During his tenure as Chair of Medicine at Duke, Stead was a central figure in implementing a novel medical school curriculum centered around a full year of research experience in medical school, in developing a productive and renowned housestaff program, and in building basic research in the Department of Medicine. His impact on academic medicine has been enormous as indicated by the 33 Stead trainees who went on to become chairs of medicine around the United States. From his experience in trying to find jobs for medical corps personnel returning from the Korean War came a major legacy of Stead, the creation of the Physician's Assistant as a health care provider and the founding of the Physician's Assistant Program at Duke University.

It may well turn out that the greatest Stead legacy will not be the programs he started or the Departments of Medicine that he built, but rather the way he thought and the way he interacted with patients, students of medicine and young doctors. Stead had, and still has, an extraordinary ability to see physical findings, hear patient concerns, and understand the problems of many types of systems. He has a unique ability to understand the essential issues of a problem, and to see a novel solution for a problem where others have not.

Very early in his career, Eugene Stead learned from Soma Weiss a deep appreciation for the biological basis of human behavior. While at Duke, Stead realized that good doctors understand that different behavior patterns are due to differences in brain structure and function, and he formulated the simple but profound notion that appreciation of the biological basis of behavior is the essence of having tolerance for human diversity.

Though now retired, Eugene Stead's thoughts are fresh and current. He foresaw the need for outcome research 30 years ago, and because of Stead and his students, the Duke Cardiovascular Data Base now leads in shaping the way that specialty is practiced. He foresaw the need for a more rational approach to the use of health care resources, the need for managed care, and for the important role of generalists and physician-extenders in health care systems. Stead foresaw the need for physician-managers in the design of health care systems, and for the central role that the computerized medical record is now playing in modern medicine. Most importantly, Stead foresaw, and now warns us against, losing the doctor-patient relationship in the age of medical technological wizardry of the 1990s.

Thus, this book is taken from what Stead has written over the past 30 years, and from a series of interviews with Eugene Stead from 1991 through 1995. The purpose of the book is to show in Stead's own words how he thinks and approaches medical problems, and what his view of being a doctor is all about. All essays and quotes in the book are from Eugene Stead, with the sources and dates listed in the final section of the book on page 177.

This book answers the question, "What does it mean to be a doctor?" in Eugene Stead's words, and provides a source of his "way of thinking" for young doctors in training both now and in years to come. One of Stead's favorite sayings on the ward, usually after a long and poorly organized presentation of what might be wrong with a patient, was "What this patient needs is a doctor!" This book tells what a doctor should be and how the doctor-patient relationship can survive and flourish—no matter what the health care system, no matter what the age.

Barton F. Haynes, MD
February, 1995

A Way of Thinking

A Primer on the Art of Being a Doctor

I

Medical Education—Learning Is a Lifelong Pursuit

*T*he method physicians select for lifelong education must give pleasure and tangible dividends because human beings will not continue a program without rewards. During medical school and residency training, the mentors ask the questions and offer praise when the answers go beyond information present in standard textbooks. Beginning doctors are puzzled by how rarely they know the answers. As superior students in the past, they always knew the answers. In time my student doctors eventually discover that Stead does not know the answers. From that moment on, learning has a different quality. Knowing what is not known is as important as knowing what is known. Physicians are ready to leave the fold when they ask searching questions about their patients and vigorously pursue the answers. The rewards include satisfaction from exercising their brains and from improving the quality of their medical practice, as well as the opportunity to hone their knowledge by teaching others.

Lifetime learners organize their practice to allow time for study, and because they enjoy using their brains, they continue to learn.

Chapter 1 ☞

Paid in Full by the Satisfactions of Each Day

E ach person must sooner or later face up to the question, "What is the purpose of life?" The answer will have a great deal to do with the way one lives and one's relationship to others. I have never had a clear understanding of the purpose of life. I have, however, defined certain limits within which I think the answer must lie and, in this way, excluded a number of possible answers which lie outside these limits.

The purpose of life can hardly lie in the past. That period of time is over and will never recur. The purpose of life can hardly be to achieve something in the future, because the future has too little reality. In some way, the purpose of life must relate to the present. The present is real and tangible. It belongs to you; it cannot be taken away from you.

The realization that the returns from living are collected each day does modify one's behavior. One is unwilling to sacrifice everything in the present for something in the future. As a doctor, I have taken care of many parents who over many years gave everything to their children with the expectation the children would repay them in future years. As the parents aged they told the children that they were all they had to live for. The children resented their parents' dependence on them and wished the parents had developed interests to supply pleasure from living independent of them.

3

Because of our[1] belief in the present, we did not give up everything for our children. We kept some time for ourselves and always spent some part of each year away from the children. What resources we had, we shared. We had our share of the free money; the children had theirs. We enjoyed our children each day and, when we put them to bed each night, the books were balanced. We had cared for them and we had enjoyed them. They owed us nothing. As the children became older, we made it clear to them that we would support them until they were able to support themselves. After that time, we would expect to see them and their children, if all of us enjoyed the venture. When they were capable of independence, we owed them nothing and they owed us nothing. We had collected our pleasures as we went and there were no debts.

Many young women and men have talked with me about their plans for the next year or years. My answers have always reflected my belief in the importance of the present. If young people are contemplating a program that they may wish they had not taken unless they achieve a particular position in some hierarchy, I advise against it. If the program pays dividends in satisfaction and pleasure while it is being pursued, they cannot lose. No matter what happens in the future, the fun of the present belongs forever to them.

I have been surprised at how rarely young doctors, engaged in planning their careers, ask the question that I judge to be of the greatest importance: "How do we plan our educational program to help us gain the greatest satisfaction out of each day of

---

1. *Our* refers to Gene Stead and his wife, Evelyn. Their three children are Lucy Stead Barnhill, a software engineer at IBM in Research Triangle Park, North Carolina, Nancy Stead Atwood, a hematologist/oncologist in Gainesville, Georgia, and William W. Stead, Director of Informatics and Vice-Chancellor for Health Affairs at Vanderbilt University.

our lives?" Their great concern is to become technically competent, and they assume that out of this, happiness will flow. Experience shows that this may be too simple an assessment.

Doctors cannot treat disease alone. They must care for the
patient who has the disease. Doctors who wake each morning
with zest for the adventures of the day are at peace with their
patients. They know the limits that the structure of the nervous
system puts on the behavior of persons. They do not expect all
things from all people. They can comfortably make fewer
demands on persons who, because of genetic background, unfavorable environment, ignorance, fear, or prejudice, have lower
ceilings of performance. The doctor who enjoys the day develops a high degree of tolerance for the frailties of man and enjoys
to the fullest the triumph of individuals. The course of education selected by young doctors should be one that teaches them
to enjoy the people who have the illnesses they have learned to
treat. This is the only way to assure that the work of each day
will bring true satisfaction.

To keep one's perspective on the problems of living, one
needs to have some sense of the geological time scale. The most
famous men and women of recorded history occupy very few
moments in our thoughts. How few of us spend any time thinking about Alexander the Great or Julius Caesar! Within a few
million years, all traces of them could disappear from the
thoughts of any living human. The purpose of life can hardly be
to obtain fame, because it is too impermanent. Events that add
to the enjoyment of the day may bring distinction and fame.
The achievement of fame and distinction at the expense of the
enjoyment of the day does not bring happiness.

The knowledge of the uncertainty of the future does influence the direction of one's life. Doctors know that they or anyone else may die before a new day dawns. The wise person is
not disturbed by this. They do each day what they want to do,

and if the date of their death were known to them, they would not need to change their plans. They have planned their lives with the knowledge of impermanence. If they live in the present, they need have no fear of the future.

Chapter 2 ☞

A Way of Learning

*M*y first professor of medicine was James Edgar Paullin,[1] an Atlanta internist who served as a President of the American College of Physicians as well as of the American Medical Association. Two mornings a week he saw patients at Grady Hospital, taught students and residents, asked questions, and used the library. He received no money for his teaching services, but allowed his private practice fees to increase as his reputation grew throughout north Georgia and the entire South. His patients never resented his unavailability on those two mornings because, as he explained, "If I'm going to give you first-rate medical care over the years, I must have continuing medical education. I'll do two things: I'll be certain that your needs are covered by someone else when I'm not available, and I'll charge you for my educational time because you are getting the kind of service nobody else in this community can give you." The old gentleman did extraordinarily well. He was the outstanding practitioner in the state; he gave first-rate care; and he died with an estate I wouldn't mind having.

In Boston, Sam Levine, a distinguished cardiologist, followed

---

1. James Edgar Paullin was Dr. Stead's first mentor and was professor of Medicine at Emory University School of Medicine in Atlanta, Georgia. (see Chapter 10).

a similar pattern, spending every morning in the Peter Bent Brigham Hospital. At one time he was paid a salary of $500, but it took him roughly 24 years to rise to that level. Then Dr. Soma Weiss[2] came along and said, "You know, I don't have much free money to pay my young people." Since I was one of the young people, I was interested in that. Soma said, "Sam, you don't really need $500, do you?" Sam said, "No, I don't need $500." So, Sam Levine lost his $500, but he still came to the Brigham Hospital every morning. He saw patients, asked questions, and tried to get answers.

Educational days not designed to pay the overhead of practice are important. They were set up as educational time required by patients' needs. Patients were asking questions the doctors were unable to answer. This was an extraordinarily efficient way to learn. I had always been surprised that people took the last year of residency training because, if you can multiply, you can see that a year distributed over seven years of practice can be used to greater advantage. There are 52 weeks in a year, and that's a lot of time. Young doctors can go into practice in the community a year earlier than they would if they took that last year of residency and say to the people, "I'm going to give you the best service over the years, but that requires that I continue my education." They can then set aside one day a week to see patients free, as a part of their continuing education for seven years. I don't care how much you teach residents in the last year of residency, they will be licked by the forgetting curve. No matter what they know at the end of the residency, they won't retain much of it seven years later. But if they learn every week, they will lick the forgetting curve.

---

2. Soma Weiss was Hersey Professor at Harvard Medical School and Physician-in-Chief at the Peter Bent Brigham Hospital in Boston, Massachusetts from 1939 to 1942 (see Chapter 11).

Not only that, they will have built in a way to control their practice. Instead of the practice running them, they will run it. Unfortunately, there are not many people who have the discipline to carry out this program. The ones who do will be the outstanding doctors in their region, state, and community. They will be learning from their patients, and they will profit from what has been discovered and rediscovered by educational experts: when you are active, it helps you lick the forgetting curve, and when you are passive, the forgetting curve always licks you.

The reason we tie learning to patients is simple. Two kinds of knowledge are stored in the nervous system: knowledge that is not used and is not freely available, and knowledge that is frequently used and is available. For example, if I keep poking at a student who knows a certain number of things, I can finally get him to put out the information. It may take a half-hour or three-quarters of an hour to get it out, because he had never before used or manipulated that material. The training and education that is directly tied to patients is designed to take stored information and mobilize it for use in a variety of contexts.

Education is added to practice when the doctor says, "I'm going to look at this problem outside my usual practice pattern. I'm going to take time to ask a series of questions that I cannot ask about every patient. I'm going to find out some of the things I don't know." Practice is really carried on by habit. Asking questions and developing answers are added educational components.

It is easier to start with the patient than it is to go to a meeting and pick up information and then take it back to the patient. I know some physicians in North Carolina who rarely go to meetings, but there's not very much you can ask them that they don't know. They have an extraordinarily simple system: they practice medicine. They learned as residents to ask relevant questions. They read *JAMA*, the *New England Journal of Medicine*, the

Lancet, and the *British Medical Journal.* They ask, "What new knowledge will be useful in my practice?" Then they use the new material in their practice. It is an effective way to learn.

The educator should primarily cultivate in the student an attitude. I have been accused of never teaching anybody anything. In general, the accusation is correct. I never lecture at Duke. I teach attitudes because everybody else is teaching facts. I ask questions like: "How do you have a good time practicing medicine and taking care of difficult patients?" Those are very fundamental questions that are not asked often enough. I spend a fair amount of time trying to answer them. I am not, however, against facts; you cannot function without them.

The formation of the correct habits and an efficient style in caring for patients is the best and most economical way to practice medicine. It is when the patient doesn't fit the pattern that you have to refer the difficult problems to someone else or take the more time-consuming thinking and learning route. Patterns are set up not only in the way you practice medicine, but in the way you finance and organize your office.

If you were to say to me, "But I don't know how best to use the time that I set aside for learning from patients," I would reply: "See some patients for education and not for production. Look at the patient's problems as if you were reading a book. During that time, ask yourself questions and, because memory is finite, write down some of them. Spend the rest of the time searching for answers to those questions. That takes discipline, but it also pays financial dividends."

Sometimes, I am asked, "Are case reports a useful device for continuing medical education?" I always reply that they have great educational value. Their preparation requires discipline. An unfinished case report is worthless. If you have ten case reports in that many subjects, you will be fun to see patients with.

I want to continue my own education for three reasons: (1) it is fun to add new material that can be converted to habit, (2) I am competitive and would like to give the best care in the community, and (3) I would like to be paid well for it. A simple, consistent program is superior to periodic elaborate programs.

I don't know how many program brochures I throw away every week. With the best of intentions, we may have created a monster. Continuing education courses are becoming a major source of income to the educational establishment, but there is little evidence that they change the behavior of doctors.

Chapter 3

Happy, Communicative and Understanding Doctors—The Roles of the "Humanities" and Bioscience

*M*any people are concerned that the extensive investment by premedical students in the physical and biological sciences will have a dehumanizing effect on them when they become practicing doctors. There is a hue and cry for courses in the humanities that, it is hoped, will produce doctors conscious of the non-technical needs of their patients. I remain skeptical. I have never observed any relationship between course content and the behavior of doctors.

I include four goals under the umbrella of general education:

1. The ability to enjoy life through a variety of inputs into the brain. Literature, art, music, drama, architecture, golf, foreign languages, running, swimming, gardening, climbing, skiing, philosophy, mathematics and science are examples. Each of us should explore a variety of areas to find those from which we can obtain real enjoyment and satisfaction. One hopes to arrive at the place where there is only a thin line between work and play.

2. Provision of a speaking and reading knowledge of history, religious thought, political science, economics, sociology and government. This is the information base which allows a citizen to be an effective force in a democracy.

3. Preparation for effective communication with persons from a variety of cultural, social, educational and economic backgrounds.

4. An understanding of the biological basis for behavior so that one can interact usefully and nondestructively with persons of different beliefs and behavior.

Prospective medical students should be urged to explore widely the world about them. Obtaining a background that allows enjoyment in a wide variety of areas takes time and effort. I have been surprised at how rarely a student asks: How can I plan my education so that I have economic security and personal enjoyment?

The importance of knowledge to become a useful citizen in our democracy is obvious and is accepted by most students. Appropriately selected courses do help in achieving the first two goals, which are the hallmarks of a well educated person—namely having fun out of life and becoming a useful citizen.

Goals three and four—effective communication and understanding differences in behavior—are not achieved by courses in the humanities. Proficiency in these areas of human interaction is much better taught as a part of bioscience. Human behavior is a mysterious chasm to those without some knowledge of the brain and the interrelationships between brain structure and function. This knowledge is not gained by courses in the humanities, which can be taught without knowledge of the biosciences.

Effective communication requires pictures, formed in the brain of one person to be transmitted to the brain of another with a minimum of distortion. The brain of the doctor may draw or select pictures to be transmitted to the patient. The doctor commonly converts the picture in his or her brain to symbols which we call words. These symbols must be reassembled by the patient into a picture. The more similar the two pictures, the better the communication.

If the brains of the sender and receiver were anatomically identical, there would be no problems in communication. But they are never identical, and the reason is inherent in the manufacture and assembly of the millions of parts that make up the brain. Kodak can make cameras that will record very similar images. The cameras are not identical but the differences are small. Brains made by biological processes have a very wide range of differences and will record a given picture in very different ways.

The distribution curves of biological data have wide bases. This results from the fact that life depends on thousands of biochemical reactions continually performed within the narrow temperature range compatible with life. These reactions are catalyzed by a large array of complex proteins acting as enzymes. These enzymes are produced by the thousands in a million different cells. It is not possible to have this many units assembling complex products without error-making. As long as the end product is compatible with life and reproduction, some of the errors are passed on to the next generation. The result is the wide diversity of biological structure and function.

A doctor's brain is unique, and the doctor has to understand that the pictures that he or she is perceiving, and his or her view of reality and fantasy, differ from those of every other human being. The patient's brain is unique, and its pictures belong only to that one brain. It is not surprising that communication between doctor and patient is difficult.

The behavior of a doctor is a function of the gross, microscopic, and molecular structure of that doctor's brain. The behavior of a patient is a function of the structure of that patient's brain. Effective communication requires that the doctor be aware of the wide differences in brain anatomy and the effects of those differences on the behavior of the patient.

The doctor as a professional assumes the responsibility for

devising effective channels of communication with patients. He or she identifies the characteristics of different patients and devises appropriate ways to transfer the picture in his or her brain to theirs. The doctor can never tell what transfers have occurred except by asking the patient to play back the picture.

Awareness of the differences in brains and the anatomical basis of behavior allows the doctor to develop an understanding of why each person is unique and cannot be remade in the image of another person. The doctor knows that the behavior of his patient has an anatomical basis and that a change in behavior requires a change in the brain itself. Experience will demonstrate that brain changing is no easy matter.

When the behavior of humankind was shrouded in mystery, tolerance for different types of behavior had no basis in science. Tolerance was something that people of good will developed, but they always were puzzled as to why other persons didn't behave like them. It was assumed that persons whose behavior was judged to be unacceptable to us and interfered with their own health and happiness could easily change their behavior in conformity to our instructions. Now that one knows that a change in the brain is a requirement for a change in behavior and that restructuring of the brain becomes more difficult with each passing day, one has to accept that people are as they are. Since each of us can at best make only small changes in behavior, tolerance of differences in behavior becomes a necessity.

The relationship between structure and function in the brain has become clearer because we are now able to make reversible changes in structure by attaching small molecules (e.g., drugs or hormones) to different areas of the brain. The fact that these changes are not identifiable by the microscope makes us aware of the many other changes that cannot be identified by the pathologist.

Wide variations in structure occur in all biological systems.

The more complex the part, the greater the diversity in structure and function. The brain is our most complex organ and therefore brains can be expected to be more different from each other than are hearts or livers. Medicine has been able to relate the changes in structure to the changes in behavior in many disease states. As yet we have made little progress in identifying the subtle anatomical changes that produce the wide diversity in brain function which we observe in persons without disease. We know that estrogenized brains differ from testosteronized brains but we do not know in detail the anatomical changes produced as these hormones attach themselves to various structures of the brain.

Neurologists have shown little interest in describing the many differences in the structures of brains which define each of us as a unique individual. It will be many years before we can define the precise arrangement of structures accounting for observed differences in behavior. We know that the differences exist because differences in function are a manifestation of differences in structure.

An understanding doctor capable of communicating with a wide variety of patients and tolerant of their differences is more likely to have become so because of a knowledge of biosciences than because of any number of courses in the humanities. Furthermore, doctors aware of the way that the brain develops and of the loss of flexibility as systems age know that our future lies with care of pregnant women and the input into brains in the early years of life. All isn't lost after the age of seven—but most is.

Chapter 4 ☞

Thinking Ward Rounds

H ow do you learn to think? One way is to practice. But what do you practice and in what setting? One way is to have ward rounds which are pointed specifically at thinking.

The learning process can be divided into the accumulation of bits of information (memory) and the movement of these bits into patterns which are new to the individual (thinking). A little reflection will make it clear that the compulsive learner is incapable of thinking. There is always another bit of information to be memorized and, if they are all learned, there is little time to rearrange the bits in original patterns. It is also clear that without any bits there is no thinking. The hardest theoretical question in educational circles is the determination of the optimum number of bits for the most effective manipulation.

Problem solving may or may not involve thinking. If one reads another person's solution to a problem, the answer is acquired through memory and no manipulation of data is achieved. If one solves a problem by the application of a known routine or formula, no thinking is required. One may obtain a solution to the problem of 98 multiplied by 7 without doing any thinking. On the other hand, solution of a problem by the rearrangement of bits of information into patterns that are new to the individual is, by definition, thinking. An attempt to solve a problem by thinking frequently serves as a stimulus to accumulating new bits of information. The addition of new bits may suddenly allow combinations of old and new memorized material to be arranged in patterns novel to the individual.

Now for thinking ward rounds. A patient is seen who has a record of nocturia. Careful questioning establishes that the patient does not have frequency from irritation of the bladder or from neurological disease, and does not have to wake to void because of a large amount of fluid imbibed shortly before bedtime or during the night. The patient, in fact, drinks normally during the day but, as recorded in the history, he excretes at night an abnormally increased volume of urine. Why is this information useful to the doctor? Identify a common denominator relating to the phenomenon of nocturia, the metabolic disturbance in thyrotoxicosis, and Cheyne-Stokes respiration associated with a greatly enlarged heart. Relate the generalization derived to the practice of medicine.

The next few minutes are spent in being certain that the problem is properly recorded. The information to be collected about nocturia, about thyrotoxicosis and about certain forms of Cheyne-Stokes breathing can be likened to the learning of arithmetic and involves mainly memory. The generalization which relates these three commonly observed clinical problems is not found in textbooks and one must convert the specific knowledge gleaned from a more perceptive look at the three syndromes into some more useful generalization. In mathematics, this would be changing from the arithmetic that $2+2=4$ to the algebraic generalization $a+b=c$.

The matter is then re-opened after several days. Several solutions may be derived but none can be achieved without thinking.

This formulation appeals to me most:

The usual sequence of drinking is well known to any beer hall keeper. He supplies large amounts of liquid and ample toilet facilities. His experience shows: beer in—beer out, no nocturia.

Our patient had uncoupled a normally well-coupled system and the uncoupling was revealed by the presence of increased water output at night without any increased fluid intake during the night.

In thyrotoxicosis, food is burned with the production of ATP. In the normal subject the burning of substances for energy is coupled to the process of phosphorylation. As ATP accumulates, the metabolic fires are banked. In thyrotoxicosis, a tightly coupled system has become uncoupled. Substrate utilization is not inhibited by normal concentrations of ATP and the amount of ATP present.

In Cheyne-Stokes respiration with a big heart, the O_2 and CO_2 concentrations of the blood entering the left heart may be greatly different from the concentrations of these gases in blood leaving by the aorta. During hyperpnea, the heart empties itself of dark blood accumulated during the previous period of apnea and at the same time fills itself with well-oxygenated blood with a low CO_2 content. The nervous system continues to respond to the unoxygenated blood with a high CO_2 content until all the black blood is gone and the heart is filled with red blood. Apnea occurs as the oxygenated blood is delivered to the nervous system, and a chemical stimulus from breathing will be absent until all the red blood is emptied from the heart. During the period of apnea, the heart is being filled from the unventilated lungs. Again a tightly coupled system relating the concentration of oxygen and CO_2 in pulmonary venous blood to the concentrations of these gases in arterial blood has become uncoupled.

We now have shown three separate disease states in which there is an uncoupling of mechanisms that are normally coupled. The generalization to be learned is that disease is a common uncoupler of coupled mechanisms, and one should bear this in mind as you work through the pathophysiologies of various disease states.

The goal of such an exercise is to improve the ability to think. Exercises related to patient care must be devised which involve thinking. The student deserves concrete illustration of thinking processes. Thinking ward rounds are useful.

Chapter 5 ☞

Preparation for Practice

T he medical profession is made up of different people. Each of these people has his best fit with his environment— physical, social and intellectual. No one school can be all things to all students. The men and women entering the medical profession will continue to have a large table from which to select, and schools will continue to have an individual flavor. Part-time faculty will play a larger role in some places than in others.

Many people believe that the internship and residency are designed as a period of supervised practice and that, during this period of supervised work, residents should be exposed to every clinical problem they will ever have to solve. Those with this philosophy structure their programs so that the residency experience is as much like practice as possible.

I have always looked on the residency years as preparation for the continuing education which should take place during practice, and I structured our program at Duke to be as unlike practice as possible. I do believe that the best residency primarily prepares for tomorrow. I am more interested in developing the ability to learn from each new situation than I am in the catholic covering of all clinical experiences. I am concerned with the learning of the language that will be used tomorrow, even though the words and concepts are not those actually used in clinical practice today. I am content to leave a large area to be filled in during those exciting early years in practice. I have no objection to the fact that our residents going into a new community have to ask the advice and help of people already established in the community. The young doctors do bring in the educational background for the medicine of tomorrow, and the established practitioner does provide them with much useful information on the practice of today. I am comfortable in defending this position because I have enough of my students at work in the field to be certain that what sounds good in theory also works in practice.

In our medical school I always assumed that our graduates will take care of both sick and well people. No amount of research aptitude or interest expressed by the doctor in training persuades us that he will not eventually doctor. The rewards, emotional and intellectual, of doctoring are too high. To be effective, physicians must be able to give of themselves without resentment. Patients must be free to make demands on physicians when patients are socially least attractive. To do this, physicians must have developed an interest in and knowledge of human behavior. They must be as knowledgeable about integrated human behavior as they are about the biochemical and physiologic processes going on in each of the parts. Physicians must know the biological substrate (people) in which discrete disease processes operate. They must be able to take care of patients regardless of the disease they develop. They must have due regard for the problems that diseases produce in the patient, in the family, and in the community. A doctor's attention must be directed toward avoiding scars in the living as well as helping the dying.

Once physicians appreciate the complexity of medicine and have learned both the thrills and difficulties of learning in a system of multiple, ill-characterized variables (a patient), they are ready to complete their education. If they wish to specialize, they should feed back into the areas of basic biology that underlie their specialty. They should spend a minimal amount of time in learning the clinical lore of the specialty. They need only enough to establish a flow of patients. The best specialists are made by practice, not by training.

The social patterns and economic base of medicine are in a state of flux. The future will certainly develop new patterns. In time, the entire history of people will be recorded as it happens. The record will begin with observations on the fetus made during pregnancy. The details of the delivery and of the first four years of life will be entered by the attending physician. A preschool examination will be part of the educational program for mother and child. The record will be updated at regular intervals and a large part of the training of the child in biology and sociology will center around his own personal history. New information will be added at the time of employment, marriage and on any visit to health personnel. Examination of blood, urine, stool, heart, lungs, vaginal secretion and breasts will be automated, and the unit cost of each determination will be very low. Information on economic status, social development, natural aptitudes and psychological development will be a part of the record. These data will be collected for more accurate subgrouping of patients for preventive as well as curative medicine.

All physicians can have a role in these projections into the future. In our medical centers, the full-time teachers are apt to take the lead not because they are brighter or more capable, but because they are paid in such a way that they have the leisure time for thinking.

Great teachers will come from all areas of the profession. All will have to face one problem, namely, that it is impossible to remain the best in any area of medicine for very long. The world does belong to the young, and my chief residents were tough competition for any professor, part-time or full-time. The secret of success is to devise a social system which allows for change.

The only thing you know for certain about a new faculty member is that he or she will change. You do not know the direction or rate of change, but you know that change will occur. The social system of the university should accept the challenge of this uncertainty and allow its faculty to live many different lives. The most common error is for the doctor to keep on doing at the age 50 what he or she was doing at the age of 30. For the majority of teachers, the real excitement wanes after 15 years. They should pass the torch to the youngsters and move on to other areas of responsibility in the school or community. Social systems created by biologists should be flexible. We should enjoy the young—not compete with them. The young should gain responsibility while they have the drive and enthusiasm to enjoy it. In this way the profession will more effectively mold the lives of people.

Chapter 6 ☞

Daniel in the Lion's Den: A Generalist among Specialists

*W*hat are generalists? By definition, they are not specialists and therefore are dependent on the help of many specialists for precise information at the cutting edge of the various specialties. Specialists go to meetings and read books in which most of the material presented is already known to them. They always carefully examine the titles of papers to be presented at meetings and the credentials of the persons presenting them, to protect themselves against wasting their time listening to things that may not relate to their specialty. Generalists set aside a portion of time for reading and listening. They explore areas in which they only in part understand the language. They rarely attend sessions where they already know most of the material.

The chief resident at Duke is a bright young doctor who is responsible for caring for patients who are seen by a multitude of specialists. When the system works, and it usually does, this young generalist taps the specialists' skills and wisdom directed to the diagnosis and treatment of the disease and pushes each specialist to the limit of his knowledge, which is defined when the answers become, "I don't know," by the more humble of the lot, and, "It is not known," by the more arrogant. Our generalist resident must care for the patient with the disease as well as for the diseases that the patient has. This process requires a sifting and reorientation of the material supplied by the specialists. I suggest to each resident that they read Winston Churchill's *The Second World War.* There, you see Churchill, a superb generalist, surrounded by specialists, remaining in charge of the operation. He uses the knowledge of each specialist, integrates it into the whole, makes the necessary series of compromises, and directs the overall operation. Specialization has been at the cutting edge of most of the advances in scientific medicine, and this will continue. The problem in medical practice is how to use the strengths that specialization can direct towards disease to give effective care to patients with multiple problems that require the services of a knowledgeable doctor but do not require the services of several specialists. It is easy to throw stones in either direction. The specialist sees patients he believes are neglected because the generalist did not refer them. The generalist sees patients who have been poorly served because the specialist has concentrated on only one aspect of their problem. In the medical center, where patients are seen by specialists as part of their educational programs, the errors usually go in the direction of too little input by the generalist. Any effective generalist will not follow all the procedures and treatments recommended by the specialists. The generalist must have a strong ego and keep all orders under his or her direction. Out in the wider world of practice, where generalists can escape specialty pressures, they tend to err in the direction of making too little use of the specialist's skills.

Generalists have a more difficult time keeping their tools sharpened than do specialists. The generalist in the medical center, called upon to see problems not solved by the specialist, faces a great challenge. Because a large medical center distills out a selected group of patients from a large population composed mostly of well persons, the prevalence of unusual disease is high, and the general internist has a good chance of making a ten-strike as his mind ranges over many possibilities. These medical center generalists who use all the assets of the medical center are among the most admired medical models of our profession. The generalists out in the communities, who are responsible for the care of all the patients from which the highly selected group of patients in the medical center are drawn, have a more difficult task. The prevalence of destructive disease being low, the methods of practice suitable for the medical center will be nonproductive. Generalists faced with too low prevalence of disease may gradually lose their skills and become inept doctors.

The attitudes toward the use of antibiotics by the hospital-based infectious disease experts and the general internists in the community highlight the old true saying: "Where you stand determines what you see." The hospital-based doctor sees immunologically deficient patients who are infected by hospital organisms and who are now resistant to the more commonly used and less toxic antibiotics (nosocomial infections). He cultures the blood, all bodily orifices, and every secretion before he initiates therapy. He tests the sensitivity of any suspected pathogens to a wide spectrum of antibiotics as an aid to guiding therapy. By contrast, the doctor in the community gives his elderly patient a store of 250 mgm capsules of ampicillin. If the patient has any one of a number of symptoms—chills, fever, change in mental state, increase in respiratory rate—he takes two capsules of ampicillin orally initially and one every six hours until he reports back to the doctor or is seen by him. He puts a specimen of urine or a specimen of sputum, if he is raising any, in the icebox. If he were destined to have pneumococcal or streptococcal pneumonia, it would be aborted long before X-ray or physical signs developed. If the infection is viral, the antibiotic can be stopped within twenty-four to forty-eight hours with no harm done. If the illness turns into a more complex pattern (this happens only rarely), more complex studies are initiated as indicated.

Our infectious disease experts rail against this commonly used method of treating acute infections in the community because of their fear that it will select out antibiotic-resistant strains. In fact, most of the antibiotic strains highly resistant to antibiotics are selected out in the hospitals where the specialists work. We have to give the devil his due: the striking decrease in morbidity and/or mortality from mastoiditis, purulent sinusitis, acute staphylococcal osteomyelitis, and pneumococcal pneumonia has resulted from the prompt use of antibiotics in the communities and not from the more elaborate protocols established by infectious disease specialists in our medical centers.

Chapter 7 ≈

Evaluation of a Liberal Education by Outcomes Rather Than by Process

I t is frequently stated that a "liberal education" best prepares a person for professional education. Many persons who give lip service to the concept of "liberal education" are at a loss to define it precisely when a naive student asks, "What is a liberal education?" A short time ago, I met with a committee drawn from the faculties of the college and medical school to discuss more satisfactory ways of handling the college/medical school interfaces. Several persons used the phrase "liberal education," and, to be certain that I understood them, I asked each of them to paint a word picture that would depict the meaning of the term in a way that could be understood by the average college student. To my surprise, no one in the group was able to do this. To my way of thinking, words or phases that create no pictures in the brain of the sender cannot be expected to create meaningful pictures in the brain of the recipient. Undefined words are noise in the system rather than information. I wrote the following letter to the faculty of Duke University:

Most persons concerned with liberal education have defined it in terms of process. The student does this and that and finally emerges from his cocoon as a liberally educated person. This is the way most doctors assess the quality of medical care. If a number of procedures are done carefully, in a defined order, the quality of care is said to be good. A more realistic method of evaluation would be to see if the patient benefited and if the benefit was achieved with minimal cost to the patient in time, money, and discomfort. This way of evaluation is called "outcome evaluation." It is more difficult to obtain the data for outcome evaluation than for process evaluation, but one quickly learns that many things considered important by process evaluation have no demonstrable effects on outcomes.

There are many processes that might produce a liberally educated person, but one is never certain which of them has worked until one assesses the outcome: whether or not the process has produced an individual who exhibits the characteristics that we have decided define a liberally educated person.

The liberally educated person has the following characteristics:

1. He or she has the ability to define and complete a task within a reasonable period of time. They have learned the art of concentration. Any subject matter can be used. Latin taught in the eighth grade by a pretty, tough young lady served the purpose for me. I wanted her to admire me, and I didn't want to take too much time from my outdoor activities. I learned to concentrate.

2. They have mastered their native tongue and all information written in that language is open to them. They can and do use this medium with which to communicate with others by speech and writing. They know that there are symbolic languages—those of biology, mathematics, chemistry, physics, electronics, computers, astronomy, music et cetera—that have to be mastered if one wishes to read widely in these disciplines. In past years, a liberally educated person would have mastered Latin, Greek and one or more currently used foreign languages. With the more extensive development and use of symbolic languages and the easy availability of translations, we have accepted the reality that most of our well-educated people will not be fluent

in a foreign language. Even today, one needs to have studied another language sufficiently in depth to understand the problems of communication between people speaking different languages. We have an army of lawyers who attempt to write documents in English with only a single interpretation; the extent of the court calendar demonstrates the difficulty of this task. Any teacher who has framed a complex question to be answered by several thousand very intelligent persons has been surprised by the fact that a few students have interpreted the question in an unanticipated but logical way that differs from that of the teacher. Precise communication between persons with different native tongues is even more difficult. One of the roles of the teacher is to make clear at each point in their student's career where the student is closing out access to important information because of failure to master a particular language.

3. Liberally educated, intelligent people will know many facts, but even more important is their ability to master new content when they have need for it. The aim of education is to give freedom, and the ability to say comfortably, "I don't know," is a great freedom. Compulsive learners of facts who are made uneasy when they don't have the latest fact immediately recallable are never original thinkers. They are at the mercy of anyone who publishes a new paper. They are in the position of the famous English physician whose angina pectoris was triggered by emotions, who said that he was at the mercy of anyone who made him mad. Some help from the faculty is due students to ascertain which facts should be laid down in their brains and which facts are best kept in tables, books, and computers.

4. The liberally educated person has the ability to take old and new facts and interrelate them into new and useful designs. This rearrangement and manipulation of facts is called thinking. Every question that has a definite answer can be answered by some arrangement of memory: from brain, books, tables, com-

puters. One can encourage students to think by requiring them to answer questions that have no agreed upon answers. Most of the faculty never ask questions without definitive answers, because they put themselves at risk. The student's answers are frequently better than the professor's.

5. Liberally educated people must have some idea of the complexity of biologic systems. They must appreciate the biologic basis of heredity and know how this can be modified by environment. They must appreciate the thousands of proteins that must be manufactured by the body and the impossibility of exact duplication of all molecules composing the body. Absolute phenotypic identity is not achieved even in twins produced from the union of one egg and one sperm. They will appreciate the basis for the width of the distribution curves of all biologic materials and know that all biologic functions in the organisms are a summation of a series of these wide distribution curves. They will know that a variety of chemicals and hormones attach to parts of the brain and alter structure and behavior.

6. Liberally educated people have tolerance for their fellow-man, because they know that their own excellent behavior is the expression of the organization of the nervous system. Injure that nervous system and the individual becomes as worthless as the next non-functioning patient. Liberally educated people know that the brain is composed of reversible and irreversible elements. Education can push the system to the limits of its capability but it cannot push beyond that point. All people are born free but not equal. True tolerance is achieved when one appreciates the biologic basis that prevents all people from reaching the same heights.

7. People with a liberal education must have some knowledge of the neurologic basis of behavior beyond that which is tested when the intelligence quotient is measured. They must know that rage, hate, the Spanish Inquisition, war, prejudice,

visual imagery, appreciation of music and the arts, and love are functions of parts of the brain not necessarily developing in parallel with those functions tested by college preparatory boards.

8. They must know the difficulties created by problems of communication between people. Each retina and brain being different, the end result of any stimulus is different. We know this from conceptual considerations; the only question is how great is the difference. Once we know that our perceptions are unique to ourselves, we have less difficulty in understanding human behavior.

9. Liberally educated people have learned the complexity of social and economic problems where the variables form a network, and one cannot precisely predict the results of changing any part of the system. They know that the complexity of the aggregates of people into families, groups, and societies is infinitely greater than the complexity of a single organism. They do not suggest simplistic solutions for complex issues.

10. Liberally educated people have a knowledge of history of their own society and an appreciation of the changes produced in the brain by socialization, including culture, religion, and other systems of belief. They appreciate the tremendous force of religious belief, and know that religious wars will continue to be fought. They have some knowledge of anthropology and the variations in behavior in different cultures. They are aware of the similarities and differences between the great religions.

11. People with a liberal education have discovered the joy of learning and continue to learn for enjoyment until their brains fail. Any area in which they have language competence is open to them, and their intellectual explorations will range far and wide.

I will leave it to the reader to decide whether our high schools and colleges have developed processes capable of producing a large number of liberally educated persons. I am skeptical that rigid programs designed to produce the highest grades on multiple choice examinations are very effective. I am concerned that our people at a young age are introduced into a very competitive system in which progression is dependent on high grades, the achievement of which may stifle individualism. The students entering medical school seem to have done too few things simply because they wanted to.

Chapter 8 ≈

Education in Medical School

*T*here has never been general agreement on the time to begin one's professional education. My own solution is to admit the students to medical school when they say they are no longer enjoying college and have the language competence in English, mathematics, computer science, chemistry, physics, and electronics considered essential by the medical faculty for mastering the material presented in medical school. The need for the colleges to keep premedical students enrolled for the tuition they bring in during the years required to attain the undergraduate degree is the greatest opposing force. As a young dean of the Emory University Medical School, I needed only one meeting with the college president to learn this simple but important fact of college financing. I have always been willing to leave out any portion of the college or medical school curricula provided that the time was saved for use at a later date. It is pointless to try to protect the individual from the need to learn after graduation by insisting that he learn a tremendous amount of what at this point in time seems to the student to be useless knowledge. It is better to leave out two years of college completely than to use these two years poorly. The concept of profitable "leaving out" and placing unused time in a bank for later use is so difficult for many people to grasp that I want to restate it. You can leave out of the curriculum anything that you want to leave out as long as

37

you also leave free the time that would normally have been invested in that area. One can take the work at a later date if he has saved the time created by "leaving out."

The role of the basic science faculty in the medical school has never been settled. The argument that they teach facts that the student must learn in one year in order to practice medicine six to ten years later is difficult to sustain. The characteristics of the "forgetting curve," the very few facts learned in Year 1 that the doctor can recall in his first year in practice, and the difference in the content taught freshman medical students six to eight years later indicate that the content of the basic science years is not very important. In the instruction of medical students, the real uses of the basic science faculty are to reinforce the liberal education that, one hopes, the student acquired in college, to encourage greater language competence among the students, and to show how various disciplines approach the solution of problems. The basic science faculty are not there to stuff the heads of medical students with innumerable facts that will be forgotten as soon as they pass Part 1 of the National Boards. They are there to give joy to the learning, to reinforce patterns of satisfaction gained from intellectual effort, and to create a research environment that brings doctors back to their basic science laboratories after they discover how frequently the unknown prevents useful clinical activity. In all honesty, I cannot identify any particular content that the basic science faculty has to teach to allow a doctor to practice medicine. It is obviously absurd to have the physiology department teach the student how to measure the arterial blood pressure in class when the practicing doctor does it many times each day.

Why does the basic science faculty not relax and gain the excitement that comes from meaningful intellectual interchange between faculty and student? I've puzzled over this for many years. The most obvious answer is that the basic science instructors do not know what information the doctor needs to practice medicine successfully and are unaware of the many inputs into the doctor's education before the doctor finishes residency. Alas, I'm afraid the real reason lies closer to the pocketbook. Medical schools support their basic scientists in terms of salary, space, and equipment beyond the level of support usually found in graduate schools unconnected to medical schools. If the facts taught in years 1 and 2 are accepted as not being essential to medical practice, some parsimonious dean might begin to eliminate the basic science instruction. I, for one, react in the opposite way. If the basic science faculty would send me students interested and knowledgeable about how to learn and eager to find additional intellectual challenges, I'd vote to double their salaries. It is in the role of stuffers of heads with facts that they seem overpaid.

I have already stated that the most important single function of the educational system is to give the student the ability to read all the relevant books. I doubt that once the student has language competence he profits by reading books that he doesn't want to read. The continual reading of books and the range of subjects covered after language competence is achieved depends largely upon the innate characteristics of the student and is only to a minor extent modified by education and further training.

Some medical students and doctors have a broad interest in medicine and biology, and others have narrow interests. The range of interest depends predominantly on the things that have molded their nervous systems long before they enter medical school and not upon their training. When two assistant residents share the same ward, each is responsible for roughly one-half of the patients. One assistant resident knows all his or her patients in detail but has a working knowledge of the problems of the patients belonging to the other assistant resident and keeps up with their progress. When the second assistant resident, equally intelligent, comes to a patient for whom he or she is not administratively responsible, he says, "This patient belongs to the other resident and I know nothing about him." These attitudes will remain with these two doctors throughout their lives and will be little changed by further education. Experience shows that selection for desired qualities at the age of twenty-plus years is a much more effective tool than training.

I had the opportunity to test out the value of selection during the twenty-six years that I held the power of appointments in departments of medicine—five years at Emory and twenty-one at Duke. I agreed with Osler's[1] statement that the magic word was work, and I was never attracted to the potentially brilliant person who might have performed but usually didn't. I baited my trap by establishing the reputation that the medical services at Emory and later at Duke were by far the most demanding of any in the world, and that only a few iron men and women could survive. I never had any interest in what the incoming intern said he wanted to do. After all, why be young except to sample a number of delicacies before making a final choice? Community specialty or general practice, academic clinical medicine, teaching and research in basic sciences, administrative medicine, military medicine were all equally acceptable outcomes. The only requirement was excellence in the pathways selected and the ability to complete the day's work. Most of the persons who entered our trap were fabulous performers. If not, they were unhappy and soon left. Emory and Duke medical interns, residents, and faculty have had an impact on the medical

---

1. Sir William Osler (1849–1919) was professor of Medicine at McGill University (1874–1884), the University of Pennsylvania (1884–1889) and Johns Hopkins University (1889–1904). Osler was Regius Professor of Medicine at Oxford in 1904. At Johns Hopkins, Osler promoted the scientific method of teaching internal medicine that played a significant role in changing American medicine.

scene far beyond that predicted by a numerical count of the output. During my active years, a number of persons visited my department to learn the secret of our success. I did nothing except enjoy the achievements of the group. The educational program had nothing special except my own conviction that the faculty could more easily impede progress than facilitate it. We could and did give honor to persons who achieved. We knew that the achievements were the result of the efforts of the individual and not of our inputs.

I am interested in the ease with which rumor is accepted by students and interns and young people in general. If the service had been as difficult as rumor said, and if we had killed off successive groups of young people each year, we could never have staffed the service. What I would call "reality testing of hearsay" is not a common occupation of the young, be they medical students, interns, residents, or young faculty members. Be that as it may, the rumor market gave us an excellent method of selecting performers. Some of the faculty regretted the bright nonperformers who never came to us. I never did.

During my career I have taught many young men and women to care for diseases that occur in young, middle-aged, and old people. I have been less successful in teaching doctors to care for the persons who have the diseases. I have difficulty even today in identifying doctors who are interested in caring for persons who have complaints that will not be removed by drugs or procedures. I have observed that the doctors who are primarily interested in the diseases eventually become bored with the practice of medicine. Our knowledge of basic processes in any area is shallow, and new information that is clinically relevant to the large majority of our patients comes slowly. After many repetitions, one performs the things related to the diseases by habit. Intellectual excitement rarely dominates the day's work. The persons who have the disease come in innumerable variations with all the drama—tragedy and comedy—that characterizes human existence. The doctor has each day wells of information about people and their lives that exceed those available to Shakespeare. The drama of human existence is ever before us. Disease and its effects are one part of the drama, but influences from chromosomes, the womb, culture, beliefs, education, religion, money, hate, fear, love, and ambition are all at play. Histories are not summations of positive findings from a check list. Doctors who do not sell their birthrights to technology and live in the excitement of the day will never find practice dull. Their conversations will be about people and their problems and not about the stock market, income taxes, and real estate deals.

Over the years, I have cared for many doctors' wives, technicians, and nurses. In many instances I have had the problem of persuading the patients that I wanted to take care of them and was glad they were not desperately ill and afflicted with nontreatable, bizarre, and unusual illnesses. The more normal the body and the more the symptoms were caused by environmental factors, the better the outlook and the happier Dr. Stead. I have been careful not to ridicule or deprecate my patients. I do not have good and bad patients. I have patients with simple problems and patients with difficult problems. When the results are poor, I am at fault—not the patient. When the patient comes to me he discharges his responsibility. I am the professional, and I cannot blame my inadequacies on the person who has entrusted himself to my care. My advice to my younger colleagues is to guard their speech and let every person they come in contact with know of their concerned and kindly feelings toward persons unfortunate enough to need to seek medical care from them. Leave your hostilities to the tennis court or the wood pile.

Chapter 9 ☞

Physicians—Past and Future

P hysicians have a number of functions in our society. They diagnose and treat illness, they attempt to prevent disease, they do biomedical research, and they plan and manage systems to deliver health care.

Medical schools have structured their educational programs to select and educate persons who are primarily interested in the care of the individual patient. This is the traditional and best understood function of the physician. It is the function that is best supported by the mathematics, chemistry, and physics required of the premedical student and by the basic sciences currently required in medical school. Let us analyze the way in which physicians go about the diagnosis and treatment of disease and observe how they use the material they learn in school.

The Traditional Physicians

Doctors are trained to maximize the performance of persons during the longest possible period of time. They identify the existing structure of the body at any one point in time and, on the basis of their knowledge, advise the person how best to handle his or her body to obtain maximal performance at minimal discomfort. In order to perform this function, the physician must divide people into various subgroups. The more precise the sub-

43

grouping, the more relevant is the advice of the physician.

A small amount of general advice is useful to the population at large and can be given without the physician's becoming involved in subgrouping. For example, all people should avoid the guillotine because it severs the head of those in all subgroups; bullets piercing the brain stem kill all persons, falls above a certain height are always fatal.

The more common situation where a physician is useful does involve subgrouping. Persons who are colorblind are separated from those who are not; those in the subgroup who differ from other people because the appendix is inflamed are identified; those who do not learn what the average person learns from given social situations are placed in a separate subgroup; those with glucose-6-phosphate dehydrogenase (G6PD) deficiency are separated from those with no deficiency; the agammaglobulinemic patients are separated from those with normal gamma globulin; the patient with a cold belongs to a subgroup separated from those without colds.

There are no two persons who are identical at a single point in time. Therefore, in the last analysis, every person belongs to his own subgroup. At the present state of our knowledge, we would gain nothing by attempting to write a complete description of each person. The differences which we know exist between two very similar persons who are functioning well in our society may not at this point in time be important enough to catalog. A subgroup that appears irrelevant at one time may be very relevant at another. For many years, physicians carried Rh-positive and Rh-negative mothers in the same subgroup before subgrouping them appropriately.

Persons have some subgrouping characteristics that last during a lifetime. As the body forms, matures, and ages, it is in continual interaction with its environment. Each interaction with its environment creates a difference which may be permanent or which may be reversible. Thus, some subgrouping characteristics are transient, lasting only microseconds.

For the purpose of clinical practice, the physician recognizes three primary types of subgroups.

1. The first type of subgroups are those to which patients belong during long periods of time and where the distinguishing characteristics are built into the system by genetic markers or by influences occurring before full maturation of the organism. Examples of this type of subgrouping are hemophilia, congenital malformations due to rubella, alteration in the brain from malnutrition, fluoride impregnation of teeth, Marfan's syndrome, G6PD deficiency, and differences in fingerprints.

2. The second type of subgroups are made up of persons exposed to an environmental stimulus of the required strength and timing to cause temporary or permanent change in the organism. For example, one of two identical twins may develop pneumonia. The exposure of one twin to the right combination of environmental influences, plus the right concentration of pneumococci, caused pneumonia. Disease imposed from the outside created a new subgroup for one of the twins. These subgroups created by environmental influences may be easily reversible, as in the common cold; they may be made more reversible by treatment, as in the pneumococcal pneumonia; or they may last many years either with or without treatment, as in tuberculosis.

3. The third type of subgroup is produced by the interaction between permanent markers and environmental influences (physical stimuli, chemical interactions, or infection). The person with cystic fibrosis is unusually liable to infection; the man with multiple myeloma has more than his share of pneumococcal infection; the blind woman has more problems with trauma; the person who makes peculiar or imperfect imprints in the central nervous system has more trouble with society.

Physicians know that continual change goes on in all their patients. The molecular structure of the body fluctuates continually: the woman is different during pregnancy and during the menstrual period; the structure of a man asleep is different from that of the same man awake—the amount of corticosteroid is different in the morning than in the evening; a woman running is very different from the same woman sitting; a high carbohydrate diet and a high fat diet will cause a marked difference in the concentrations and activities of many enzymes in the liver; the same man quarreling with his wife, having sexual intercourse, or giving a lecture to a group of his peers will be composed of different molecules. Reversible changes may occur from things outside the body, or they may come from changes within the body by bacteria or viruses that normally inhabit the body, by activities of organs such as the continually beating heart or by internally generated activity within the nervous system or other organs.

Once physicians have identified the subgroup or subgroups to which the patient belongs, they may do one of several things:

1. They may have a method of changing the body so that the patient moves from one subgroup to another: a child with a patent ductus arteriosus may be removed from that subgroup by having the ductus ligated; a patient with pernicious anemia may be moved from the category of a person with too little vitamin B_{12} into the group with an adequate supply of B_{12}. In this instance, the original defect causing the B_{12} deficiency may, of course, persist.

2. They may find that a combination of circumstances has affected an otherwise normal body and that things will right themselves if the body is supported either by general measures or by treatment directed toward removing the offending agent: children with mumps recover with only general support; patients with meningococcal meningitis require therapy directed at limit-

ing the growth of the meningococcus; a patient with tachycardia or impending thyrotoxicosis may revert to normal if the interpersonal conflict initiating the disturbance can be removed or controlled; the patient with menopausal symptoms may recover as her body adjusts to the change in hormones.

3. Physicians may identify a person as belonging to a particular subgroup if the patient is harmed by certain stimuli that are well tolerated by the general population. The role here of the physician is to properly identify the subgroup, and to devise ways to help the patient arrange his life in a way that would spare him the penalties usually belonging to his particular subgroup. This is a physician's most important activity.

Proper subgrouping, acceptance of the subgroups by patients, special input for selective education, avoidance of situations which show the subgroup at its worst, and enhancement of situations which are advantageous to the subgroup are often repeated elements in medical practice. A musical composition may have infinite variability, but it may be played on the same instrument. The medical drama has infinite variability, but its general form and arrangement are more fixed than the classical Greek play.

Clinicians have the same opportunity as the chemist; they can use tests from many disciplines; they can watch their patient undergoing chromatography in the fluid of existence. Like runs alike; persons belonging to different subgroups run differently. Physicians do not have to be confined to the usual tests written down in medical texts. They can use many frames of testing to determine likeness and nonlikeness.

The most difficult problem facing physicians is to determine why their patient became better, remained unchanged, or became worse. If the patient has improved, was the fundamental defect changed or did the patient improve because of the familiar sequence of acceptance, special education, and avoidance? In either case, we would have to equate improvement with change. The change may have been in the central nervous system, in the lung, in the immunological system, or in any part of the body that has maintained the ability to undergo reversible change. We equate this reversible change in the central nervous system with education and training. It must be a change in structure, although we have not identified either the type of structural change or its location.

What are the limits of reversible change? They clearly define the limits of most doctoring. They no longer define the final limits because artificial organs and transplantation may operate beyond the previously accepted limits of reversible change. The advent of modern drug therapy has shown that the limits of reversible change are greater than we once thought.

I have, of course, included the psychiatrist in my references to clinicians. Psychiatrists are physicians trained to detect differences in subgroups on the basis of the behavior of the person. Traditionally, their subgroups are determined by the behavior of feelings, thoughts, ideas, and motivations, behaviors that are clearly embedded in and derived from the structure of the central nervous system. Psychiatrists use the traditional methods of making subgroups and attempting to improve the patient by (a) moving him to another subgroup by drug or shock therapy, or (b) making him perform better in the original subgroup by the familiar sequence of acceptance, avoidance and special education. Psychiatry differs from other clinical activities only in that, somewhat more frequently, structural arrangements underlying thinking, idea formation, habit patterns, feeling states, and motivation have not been anatomically well defined. We do not yet have an anatomical and biochemical definition to fit each clinical subgroup. Most subgroups in other disciplines were first defined by differences in clinical behavior and, at a later date, by definitive anatomical, biochemical, and pathological differences. The subgroups of psychiatry are as tightly tied to structure as are all other subgroups.

All sciences that allow us to characterize people, to subgroup them accurately, to permit us to move them from one subgroup to another or to protect them from harm while they remain within their subgroup are of equal interest to medicine. To date, we have used surgery, anatomy, microbiology, genetics, immunology, pathology, and physiology to the greatest extent. Clinical psychology and psychiatry are contributing to our knowledge of subgroups within the nervous system; bioengineering is becoming increasingly important; computers let us handle more subgroups; cardiac pacemakers and artificial kidneys let us move patients from one subgroup to another. Economics, business management, systems engineering, political science, and sociology are little used in the education of the traditional doctor because they serve no subgrouping function.

The Managing Physician

Physicians educated in the traditional way give excellent services to their patients. They are in great demand and work a long day. They are frustrated because the methods of collecting data and analyzing it for subgrouping purposes—which were ideal during their educational years—are not useful to them when they have to handle a large quantity of work. They do not know how to handle large masses of information; they are not knowledgeable about computers; they have had no experience in systems engineering; they have never devised any combinations of men and machines to give them an effective clinical support system; they do not know how to arrange for a flow of services from the community back to their office with the use of community aides, public health nurses, and physician's assistants. They know that the demands of their patients have taken all the time out of their day, and they don't know how to recreate time.

Medical schools are just now facing up to the fact that they need physicians trained in both management and medicine. When we say that premedical education should include more of the information sciences, business administration, economics, sociology, and systems engineering, we are not thinking of the traditional physician, but we are expressing our conviction that we need managing physicians.

Many people believe that persons other than physicians should serve the management function and that the physician should continue to be educated to work entirely with the individual person. This is the way the rest of our society is organized. Why not medicine? The physician does deal with matters of life and death. He can paralyze many needed changes because of his statement, "If you do that, x number of patients will die." The manager who is not a physician has no way of knowing whether the statement is true or false. Part of the management of patients is dictated by knowledge and understanding of the disease processes. A large part of the management is empirical and can be done in a variety of ways. The manager who is not a physician never knows which part is science and which part is custom. The language of medicine imposes a great barrier between the physician and other persons. It is a revealing experience to watch a group of physicians interact with computer scientists. The need for physicians who are also computer scientists comes through loud and clear.

I think no one can settle by discussion whether medical schools should train managerial physicians. I believe that several medical schools should undertake this experiment and produce physicians interested and knowledgeable about the managerial, informational, and social sciences—a physician who can either practice medicine or engage in the design and operation of health care systems. At the present time we are producing physician-scientists who can either practice medicine or engage in biomedical research. Our new product would be a physician-manager, who would either practice medicine or manage portions of the health care system.

The social, economic, political, and organizational problems which have to be solved before we can evolve satisfactory patterns for the delivery of health care are as difficult as those which had to be solved before the medical scientists could develop polio vaccines or open-heart surgery. We believe that well-motivated students who have not prepared themselves for solving these difficult problems will not have any major effect on health care systems. Medical students working in their spare time in neighborhood health clinics will find out how hard the problems really are; they will not come up with any viable solutions.

In the past, it was considered impractical to train an appreciable number of physicians for both management and the delivery of personal health services, because it was assumed that the two programs would have to be additive. The student had to jump all the bioscience hurdles before he could become a doctor, and he received no credit for any work towards the MD degree outside the traditional bioscience base. Our observations indicate that a considerable amount of bioscience can be replaced by other material without reducing the quality of patient care given by the physician. The managerial sciences will make as satisfactory a base as the biosciences for the general development of the physician's brain. To practice medicine, he has to learn only the bioscience directly applicable to the giving of personal health services. This can certainly be done in a year, leaving one year free for courses not now taught in the medical school. If he decides to become a traditional physician, he can broaden his bioscience base during his internship and residency.

The production by the medical school of physicians knowledgeable in the social and managerial sciences will require the following changes:

1. The development of the medical center and its outreach programs into the community as a laboratory for the university. This will require space in the medical center for divisions of the departments of economics, business administration, systems engineering, computer science, and sociology, where undergraduate medical students, interns, residents, and graduate students from the new disciplines work together on health problems. The faculty of the new divisions will need to learn the culture of the health area and the peculiarities of the ill. Creation of these divisions outside the heart of the medical center will result in no excitement and no change within it.

2. Acceptance of the members of the new divisions on the admission, curriculum, and promotion committees.

3. Admission of a different type of student. The medical schools have depended nearly entirely on the biosciences to prepare their students for the practice of clinical medicine. Students must jump these hurdles before they can enter the clinical arena. If students are well prepared in bioscience, they will find the preclinical work intellectually rewarding, and they will be prepared for a career as medical scientists or as practicing physicians. If they are not well prepared in biosciences, students will pass their preclinical work by memorizing and, a few years later, will be practicing medicine with little knowledge of bioscience. Students with real aptitudes in information sciences, sociology, systems engineering, economics, and business administration usually reject medical school because they do not want to spend two years memorizing facts that they will later make little use of. All medical schools have given lip service to admitting students with strengths other than those in bioscience but, when the chips are down, they have not modified their bioscience hurdles.

4. The agreement that no one department can determine that a student cannot be a physician.

A physician who in college was interested in the social and

managerial sciences and who had one year of his medical work in these areas would be prepared to (a) become an intern and resident and practice medicine; (b) find a job in the health care field related to some phase of management; and (c) continue in graduate school and develop research capabilities in health-related economics, sociology, systems engineering, business management, computer science, and data processing and retrieval.

Most medical schools intend to increase the number of students per class. In a few schools, the number of students equal to the present incoming class could continue to be selected on the basis of their competence and interest in bioscience, and the additional students admitted as enrollment is expanded could be selected on the basis of their competence and interest in the social, managerial, and information sciences.

The successful development of this program in a few American medical schools can have far-reaching effects on health care systems in all parts of the world. The rate of development of more effective man-machine systems for the delivery of health care will always be limited by the number of imaginative and capable leaders that are produced. Medical schools in emerging countries will in part pattern themselves on the models they find in this country. The bioscience model is a good one for the training of the physician who will give personal health services. It is a poor one for the development of physicians to manage health care systems.

II

Role Models

Jack Myers[1] frequently said that much clinical learning could be summarized by the statement: any positive observation has greater weight than any negative observation. If a marble is found in a room, that is a positive observation and, in general, means that the room did contain a marble. If the doctor finds no marble on searching the room, it may mean that there is no marble there, but many times it will mean that the doctor is not good at finding marbles.

---

1. Jack Myers was in Dr. Stead's department at Emory (1942–1947) and at Duke (1947–1955), and was Chief of Medicine at the University of Pittsburgh from 1955 to 1970 (see chapter 12).

Chapter 10 ⌒

My Mentors

I am not wise enough to bring to you the philosophies of the ages. I can bring to you the philosophy that has guided me in my own development. This philosophy has been developed over the years by contact with many mentors, but in a great measure it has resulted from the various Chiefs under whom I have worked. I would like to share with you some of the things which they have taught me.

My first Professor of Medicine was Dr. James Edgar Paullin of Atlanta. He was also our family doctor. He first showed me in his work that the family doctor of the future was going to be the intelligent, interested internist. He made home calls rarely, but he knew every member of my family, and no medical attention was ever sought without first reviewing the problem with him. Dr. Paullin showed me that the community was interested in the growth of its doctors. Every Tuesday and Wednesday morning he was at Grady Hospital (the city hospital of Atlanta and teaching hospital of Emory Medical School). His private patients respected his desire for continued growth as a doctor and never begrudged him this time. He was interested in medical politics and repeatedly demonstrated that all human group endeavor involves some type of political activity. He was a medical politician in the best sense of the word and all of American medicine profited by his broad interests.

My second chief was Henry Asbury Christian.[1] Under his guidance the Peter Bent Brigham medical resident staff developed many leaders in medicine. The atmosphere of the Brigham was one that gave honor to scholarship. There I first learned that, just as many people liked to fish or play golf, I liked to work with my head. Dr. Christian was successful in the development of leaders because he fostered in his residents a willingness to take the initiative. His attitude was not that the Brigham service was good because of the senior staff, but that it was good in spite of the senior staff. He relied heavily on the fact that he had pulled into his net many bright residents from all sections of the country, and he expected them to produce. I have never seen residents more conscious of their ability to learn for themselves than those resident groups assembled by Uncle Henry.

My third chief was Elliot Cutler,[2] under whom I served a 16-month surgical internship. He was loved and honored by all of his staff—even the lowly intern. On his service I discovered how hard surgeons work, and I learned that those long hours in the operating room use up the time which the internist loves to spend talking with his patients and teaching.

My fourth chief was Marion Blankenhorn[3] of Cincinnati. He gave to me my basic interest in clinical observation. Under his guidance, the history and physical examination came alive. His teaching centered around the patient and he destroyed once and for all my interest in dry clinics. He gave his resident a very free hand in running the service, and from him I learned not

---

1. Henry Asbury Christian was Professor of Medicine at the Peter Bent Brigham Hospital in Boston, Massachusetts from 1908–1939.

2. Elliot Cutler was Professor of Surgery at the Peter Bent Brigham Hospital.

3. Marion Blankenhorn was Professor of Medicine at the University of Cincinnati Medical Center.

only to do my own work but how to get other people to work.

My fifth and last chief was Soma Weiss.[4] By that time, the clay was better worked and more ready for the molding, and Soma taught me many things. He demonstrated the importance of the undergraduate student in our own learning. Repeated efforts to explain to the student the basic mechanisms of health and disease kept before us the extent of our own ignorance and made us examine critically the premises on which we based our glibly quoted clinical aphorisms. We learned the importance of appreciating what is not known. I have never ceased to drink from this well of undergraduate naiveté and skepticism.

The same use of teaching as a learning device was employed with the resident staff. Every intern and resident taught students, not because there was no other way to teach the student but because of the learning value to the resident group.

From Soma I learned the importance of keeping down artificial barriers which interfere with learning. Whoever knew the most about the problem—be he second-year student, instructor or visitor—was cock-of-the-walk for the moment. Soma achieved remarkable give and take with everyone contributing to the learning pot and everyone taking knowledge back out. He realized that the goal of the medical student was the opportunity for the correlation and consolidation of his knowledge which can be achieved only in the fourth year. He was never willing to sacrifice that period of high learning for the fourth-year student, stimulated to its fullest by an alert resident staff, for ease of operation of the outpatient clinic. The student was a doctor taking care of his patient under supervision. Therefore, as a doctor, therapeutic and diagnostic decisions could be made only with the student present. This made joint ward rounds with students, interns and residents imperative and greatly increased the cohesiveness of the group.

---

4. For a more detailed discussion of Soma Weiss see Chapter 11.

Soma never forgot that the function of a university service was to train students, and the output of research was always secondary to this main objective. He carried on research with the resident staff for its effect on their thinking. Research with the older staff was a means of keeping their minds alert and their teaching interesting.

In the laboratory, Soma taught us the value of always carrying out some observations each day on a patient. Even if the experimental procedure proved useless, we always learned something from the patient. He was never uneasy about development of the specialized knowledge of the physicist, the biochemist, or the physiologist. He always believed that doctors with sound clinical training who spent time in learning the ways of sick patients could hold their own in the research field. He emphasized the time and hard work that went into the understanding of patients and the mechanisms of diseases, and never begrudged the years necessary for the development of clinical skills.

He taught us the value of not giving up too easily, and yet he kept us from beating our heads against a stone wall on a problem for which methods then known were inadequate. He brought new methods into the laboratory and was always searching for collateral evidence to buttress any thesis he entertained. This willingness to approach any problem from many angles accounted for the soundness of his final conclusions and for his amazing ability to write many papers with so few errors in basic concepts.

Soma maintained a great interest in the symptoms that patients presented. He realized that the learning of medicine from the practice of medicine was dependent entirely upon an accurate evaluation of the cause of the patient's complaint. A patient with heart disease who complains of shortness of breath may have congested lungs which are causing the dyspnea, or he may be short of breath from anxiety, or he may have independent lung disease. If the doctor mistakes emotional dyspnea for congestive failure, he learns nothing from treating the patient.

In his study of symptomatology, Soma appreciated the complexity of medicine in modern society. He was aware of the frequency with which multiple factors operate to produce disease and symptoms. He became interested in the mechanisms by which emotional reactions cause the patient to feel abnormal. The beautiful series of experiments carried out in his laboratory on carotid sinus fainting remain of primary importance because they demonstrate reflex ways of feeling unreal, light-headed, and even becoming unconscious. These observations were not important in curing patients with fainting by denervating the carotid sinus; they were important in demonstrating reflex mechanisms for feeling abnormal.

Soma not only knew what he wanted to do, but he knew how to get it done. He didn't rail at the political moves necessary to keep the city fathers happy. He knew that all the ruling powers were people and he enjoyed handling people. It made little difference whether they were sick folk or people with power who needed education. He showed that administration was a necessary function and could be fun in its own way.

Soma Weiss had a unique degree of interest and enthusiasm for what we did which went far beyond our professional activity. He had an understanding of our personal lives and of our hopes and ambitions. He was interested in our clinical problems and in any observation we made in the laboratory. He shared with us the thrill of those first observations which are so exciting and also so apt to be not repeatable. He enjoyed any of our little triumphs as much as he enjoyed his major ones. No wonder we worked long hours and tried to think great thoughts. Here I learned the secret of running a successful medical department: the chief must assemble about him a number of people, any one of whom can outdistance him in some field. If this can be accomplished without arousing anxiety and jealousy, there will develop an excellent department whose chief enjoys tremendous satisfaction from the growth of his staff.

Chapter 11 ☞

Soma Weiss: The Characteristics that Made Us Know He Was a Great Man

*M*ost medical teaching in 1939 was directed at describing a disease. One listed the symptoms, the signs, and the pathology. Soma Weiss listened to the patient describing how he felt and the changes in his life produced by illness. He then fastened on the major symptoms. He surveyed the fields of medicine to see how often this symptom occurred, and the many disturbances in pathophysiology that could produce the symptom.

Fainting (syncope) was a good illustration. It occurred in patients with hysteria, heart block, aortic stenosis, pulmonary hypertension, epilepsy, exsanguination, postural hypotension, pregnancy, and in a number of other states. It also accompanied many benign conditions such as the sight of blood, bad news, hyperventilation, hypoglycemia, acute infections, prolonged bed rest. It could be produced in normal subjects by combining motionless standing with sodium or amyl nitrate. Thinking physiologically about symptoms rather than textbook descriptions allowed the student to make useful bedside observations. Soma was always aware of the importance of the nervous system in health and disease. He used the cardiovascular system to demonstrate the importance of neurogenic input—particularly the carotid sinus reflex, the blood pressure and pulse rate adjustments of postural changes, and the effects of hyperventilation.

Following Soma's approach, I always carried a tray with a

water manometer during my first year at the Thorndike Memorial Laboratory. Venous pressure changes occur in a variety of physiologic and pathologic states. The information that I obtained and its use on ward rounds was different from that of the average attending physician.

Soma studied heart failure in the usual patient but extended his observations to the twenty or so less common causes of heart failure. This led to a discussion of a broad spectrum of diseases. He collected unusual manifestations of heart failure. I still have a collection of his slides showing patterns of localized pulmonary edema in left ventricular failure. These findings were commonly interpreted as pneumonia rather than heart failure. I recently collected a nickel on a bet because our residents failed to recognize this type of local edema in a man with an acute myocardial infarction.

Soma had the wisdom to listen to his young staff who described what was known about the disease. He listened to the patient and asked questions about what was not known about the disease. In the course of the discussion, Soma elected to bring back more information about certain aspects of the problem and encouraged others to explore areas that had been defined by the discussion. He created a pool of knowledge to which each contributed and from which each extracted.

Soma had the magic touch of making the day seem more meaningful. He recruited talented people because he was enjoying himself. He never questioned the fact that young men could think and contribute. Soma and Corneille Heymans, a Belgian scientist, were writing a definitive account of the carotid sinus reflex when I arrived at the Thorndike. He asked me to read it and comment. I had a number of suggestions, some good, and some showing my lack of experience. Soma reviewed my comments and discussed them with me. I knew that I was not his equal, but he made it appear that I was.

We always knew that performing well could only help us. Soma was too secure to worry about our triumphs. He enjoyed winning, but he could lose gracefully, knowing that each of his losses strengthened our ego.

After I had been at the Thorndike nine months, Soma called me to his office to tell me that he and William B. Castle were supporting a young colleague for election to the Young Turks (American Society of Clinical Investigation) that year, but that next year I would be a candidate. At the Peter Bent Brigham Hospital, Soma allowed his young team of Charles A. Janeway, John Romano, and me to assume major administrative responsibility. When he was away, I filled in for him, and he handled my doing so in a way that avoided any feelings of resentment by the senior members of the staff. He placed us on all types of programs, and listened to us practice our presentations.

It is difficult to rank Soma as a diagnostician. After all, he usually saw patients after their exposure to an energetic, knowledgeable, and alert staff. His forte was to elicit the symptoms and signs and to relate them to pathophysiology. He then looked for similar states over the spectrum of normal and abnormal physiology. He was more alert than most to the feeling states engendered by culture, education, economics, family ties, and the disease. I had the advantage of watching Soma handle the Irish politician who ran the Boston City Hospital. He never missed a trick, and he always got what he wanted.

Soma had the patience to listen to his young staff and to listen to the patient. Bedside rounds were related to the patient. A diagnosis of peptic ulcer did not result in a lecture by Soma on peptic ulcer. The discussion centered on that particular patient and was much more broadranging than a textbook presentation of peptic ulcer.

Soma's ability to read rapidly in German gave him immediate access to a wide range of knowledge. Most of us had to wait for translations, and we were usually several steps behind. He enjoyed clueing us into a broader world.

Part of his reputation as a clinician came from his Tuesday night rounds at the Boston City Hospital. He started on the eighth floor of the Medical Building with the neurology service and went down floor by floor examining any patient that the house staff wished him to see. They picked their most unusual patients, and Soma saw them with no advance preparation. After finishing the eight floors in the Medical Building, he visited the two floors of the Peabody Building, which housed the Fourth Medical Service.

It was a rich clinical experience. Soma taught the house officers on the five university services at the City Hospital[1] and they in turn kept him alert to a wide variety of ever-fascinating clinical problems. House officers, students and medical visitors went out, over this and other countries, reporting that they had attended rounds at the Boston City Hospital that were conducted by an attractive, brilliant clinician who would see difficult patients of all varieties and shed light on their problems. He spoke with a Hungarian accent, sometimes inverted the usual sequences of words, and always made the patient glad to be presented on rounds. His name was Soma Weiss, and they spread the word if you ever went to Boston, you should remember to attend the Tuesday evening rounds. No wonder that Soma became a legend before his fortieth birthday.

Soma's magnetism is well illustrated by the remarks of a physician who attended a lecture sponsored by the American College of Physicians. Soma's talk was scheduled for 9 A.M. and by the time the physician and I arrived at 9:05 there was standing room only, and Soma had begun his talk. She and I listened

---

1. The Medicine services in 1937 at Boston City Hospital were I and III, Tufts; II and IV, Harvard; and V, Boston University.

to him together, and at the end of the hour she turned to me
and said, "I came to hear Soma Weiss and was disappointed to
find a young man substituting for him. However, I don't believe
that even the famed Soma Weiss could have given a better lecture than this young man. What is his name?" I replied, "Soma
Weiss."

Chapter 12 ☞

Jack Myers and Medicine

J ack Myers'[1] and my paths first crossed on September 1, 1939, the day that Hitler bombed Poland. Paul Beeson[2] was the chief resident at the Brigham and he had an unusually attractive staff of assistant residents and interns. Jack Myers, the person who was to become the doctor's doctor, was among them. Jack had graduated from Stanford and interned in the Stanford University Hospital, then located in San Francisco. He was a protégé of Arthur Bloomfield, the professor of medicine at Stanford. Because the medical service had only a very limited number of beds, Bloomfield required his staff to extract from each patient the maximal amount of information. Bloomfield's philosophy, that a few patients carefully observed and followed were a more valuable asset than many patients seen superficially, was accepted by Myers. The extraction of maximal information from each person required a knowledge of the clinical literature and the correlation of the clinical material with the relevant portions of

---

1. Jack Myers was in Dr. Stead's department at Emory (1942-1947) and at Duke (1947-1955), and was Chief of Medicine at the University of Pittsburgh from 1955 to 1970.

2. Paul Beeson was with Dr. Stead at Emory (1942-1947) and was Physician-in-Chief, Department of Internal Medicine at Yale School of Medicine from 1952 to 1965.

basic scientific knowledge. Jack was a master of marshalling the clinical data in ways that allowed logical analysis. To this framework of tightly organized data describing the patient, he added his extensive knowledge of the literature.

Those of us at the Brigham in 1939 had no doubt that Myers would succeed Beeson as chief resident at the Brigham. In those days the chief resident lived in the hospital and was the doctor in charge when the physician-in-chief, Soma Weiss, was out of the hospital. Myers ran a tight service. There was a sense of enthusiasm and achievement in the air and his group responded to the challenge of achieving clinical excellence. If one of them could "ace" Jack Myers, his day was made. As we all know, the number of Myers wins exceeded the number of wins of the rest of his team added together. These were great days!

Myers was a member of the Brigham-Harvard army unit headed by Elliott Cutler.[3] This unit was among the first to be called into active service in World War II. In time this unit was observed to have too many persons with superior leadership qualities, and it was bled extensively. The replacements came from a wide variety of schools. It was quickly recognized that one's past experience made little difference if one came under the direction of Jack Myers. If you didn't have the habits of an excellent doctor, you soon acquired them. We had known for many years that the internship and residency were more important determinants of excellence than the medical school one attended. Service under Myers was an advanced residency and he grew a crew of strong, capable men.

Soma Weiss's death in early 1942 left the Brigham's young staff without a personal mentor. On return from the Service, Jack went to the Thorndike Memorial Laboratory at the Boston City Hospital, where his reputation as an outstanding clinician

---

3. For a discussion of Elliott Cutler see page 58.

continued to grow. Paul Beeson and I were at Emory and Grady Hospital. After several attempts, we finally persuaded Jack to come to Atlanta. By that time Jessica Lewis, who was a medical star in her own right, had joined up. Before long she became Jack's wife and began to produce young Myerses along with hematologic research data of the highest quality.

Jack, who was already interested in diseases of the liver, developed a technique for measuring splanchnic blood flow based on the fact that the liver was the principal producer of urea. He set up the methods with his usual efficiency and in short order showed that the values obtained by the urea method were in agreement with the data obtained using the bromsulphthaline method. In the course of these studies he showed that the pressure obtained through a catheter wedged in a small hepatic vein reflected the pressure in the portal vein. This discovery opened the way for a series of studies on all forms of liver disease where a knowledge of the pressure in the portal vein was an important datum for diagnosis and treatment.

In 1946 the VA Hospital in Atlanta was affiliated with Emory and a Dean's Committee was formed. Jack Myers was loaned to the VA on a half-time basis and became chief of the medical service at Lawson General Hospital. He immediately attracted a group of eager young staff and in a short period of time a sleepy VA service became an aggressive university unit.

I moved to Duke on January 1, 1947 and persuaded Jack Myers, John Hickam and Frank Engel to join me in the spring. Sam Martin, a Washington University product, who became chief resident at Duke in July 1947, always teased me and my transplanted Emory team. He said that each of us in his heart wanted to be chief resident but that we couldn't have our wish because *he* was the chief resident. Sam was right: we were all immersed in clinical medicine and weren't averse to staying in the hospital all night.

Jack Myers had a great influence with the students, residents, faculty and doctors practicing in Atlanta and Durham. He was a stern taskmaster and always demanded excellence. He was not loved by everyone but was respected by all.

Jack Myers is in his element in a clinical pathologic conference. His first performance at Duke was a masterpiece. The patient had died of an unknown, mysterious infectious disease. When analyzed by Jack, the illness became a typical and classical textbook entity. Jack announced at the end of his discussion that there was no need for an elaborate differential. There could be but one answer: tularemia. He was right. For some time thereafter the members of the Duke staff who had seen the patient during life questioned whether this knowledgeable, determined young doctor would be welcome at Duke. The answer turned out to be that he was a great asset.

There is also a Pittsburgh story about his clinical and pathology skills. The primary clinical discussant gave a brief and uninspired presentation which brought Jack to his feet. He disregarded the material discussed by the designated speaker and with no advance notice gave a polished presentation of the clinical and basic science material relevant to the patient. He concluded with an accurate summary of the findings that he expected the pathologist to demonstrate. The pathologist, a few minutes later, confirmed Jack's predictions.

Jack Myers was equally capable in other areas. *Lymphogranuloma venereum* was by this time an uncommon disease at Duke. Albert Heyman[4] who had run the venereal disease clinic at Emory was particularly knowledgeable of this illness. He happened one day to be on the ward where Jack was seeing a patient with this sexually transmitted viral infection. To his sur-

---

4. Albert Heyman, MD is Professor of Neurology at Duke University Medical Center.

prise, Jack gave a complete discussion of the problem with reference to both early and recently published material.

Jack has always had the unusual ability to present material orally which requires little or no editing to turn it into a finished manuscript. This is the result of a well-ordered mind. I have met only one other person who has this unusual ability.

At Duke, all the medical staff were required to see patients in the private diagnostic clinic. Jack's commitment was for one-half day each week; the rest of his time was reserved for teaching and research. This tying of the commitment to time rather than income has worked well in most instances, but Jack's clinical skills could not be kept under a bushel basket, and demands for his services were unusually difficult to control. The problem was solved by Jack's accepting the post of chairman of the Department of Medicine at the University of Pittsburgh School of Medicine.

Young doctors ask when it is time to leave Duke and accept a larger assignment. The answer is when the brightest young doctors at Duke want to go with you. Wallace Jensen, Gerald Rodnan, Bob Kibler, and Jape Taylor left me immediately to go with Jack Myers to Pittsburgh. Jack was ready for his own show.

It is fitting that persons interested in simulating human intelligence by computers have selected Jack Myers as the brain to be simulated—a doctor's doctor; even the computer people[5] recognize that.

---

5. The computer programs *Internist I* and *II* were designed to mirror Jack Myers' personal database in general internal medicine.

Chapter 13 ☞

The Thorndike Unit at Boston City Hospital: 1937–1939

I n the winter of 1937, Soma Weiss visited the General Hospital in Cincinnati at the invitation of Eugene Ferris. Ferris had worked with Soma at the Thorndike on the mechanisms of carotid sinus syncope (fainting). In my role as chief resident at Cincinnati General Hospital, I spent five days with Soma discussing patients. He suggested that I come to the Thorndike in the nominal role as chief resident and work with him for two years at a salary of $900 per year. I replied that, because of my own loans as a student and the helping hand I was giving my brother, I could not come for less than $1,800 per year. He said that no resident at the Thorndike had ever been paid that much. I told him not to worry: that he was the only person I was interested in working with, and that I'd be available until September when I would begin the practice of medicine in Atlanta. Some time in April, a wire came stating that the $1,800 was in hand. As of July 1, I arrived at the Thorndike.

My role as chief resident at the Thorndike was not demanding. My main responsibility was to be sure that all the lights in the building were turned off each night. I saw George Minot, the chief of the service, for a few minutes each morning. I never discovered what Dr. Minot did in his role as chief. He clearly did something, because the place ran more smoothly when he was around.

75

I had never been in a research laboratory. On July 1, with my face swollen and bandaged from contact with a squash racket, I appeared in Minot's office. He seemed not to see my traumatized face and asked politely what I wanted. When I suggested that I start work, he said that Soma was in Europe for a few months and that I could look around Boston until he returned. Having spent three years in Boston before my Cincinnati venture, this did not appeal to me. I wandered up to Soma's lab and discovered to my surprise that I had a technician. Robert Wilkins had worked in Soma's laboratory the previous two years. I asked Weiss's staff what Wilkins would have done if he had been there the first day of July. They said that Drs. Weiss and Wilkins had standardized a procedure for inducing syncope (fainting) in humans, and that Wilkins would have tested out the effects of some drug on this preparation. Weiss's technicians described the protocol, suggested the drug to be tested, told me how to set up the instruments and how to find a subject. I became operational on day one, and before Soma returned, Paul Kunkel and I had completed our first paper. I took the typed manuscript (or what I thought was a manuscript) to Marian Shorley in the Department of Medicine.

She went through it with a red pencil and told me she would correct this one atrocity but, if I did not show rapid improvement, she would never help me again. The greatly improved paper landed on William Castle's desk. He read it with care, made a number of thoughtful suggestions, and the paper was on the way to the *Journal of Clinical Investigation* for quick acceptance and publication. Life was simple in those days.

Soma returned in the early fall. What a delightful two years followed. Our laboratory was at the head of the stairs on the fourth floor. Soma's office was at the opposite end of the hall. Early each morning and late each afternoon he visited the laboratory. His invariable greeting was "What's new?" In retrospect,

I'm surprised at how often we came up with something new. Kunkel and I patterned our work so that we made some kind of observations on a human, normal or sick, each morning or afternoon. It was nearly impossible not to learn something, and sharing it with Soma was a great experience.

The Thorndike was peopled with great persons. Minot, I've already said, did not affect me directly but something in the man and in his dedication to knowledge permeated the Thorndike.

William Castle was the most original thinker of my Thorndike mentors. I first met him on the steps of the Peabody Building. A resident was describing the course of a patient with kidney disease and his projected treatment. I pointed out to him the error of his ways, and the resident defended himself by telling me that he was following Castle's instruction. I replied that I didn't believe Castle knew much about this problem. I sensed without turning around that a third person had come near enough to hear this exchange. On turning around, the newcomer said, "I'm Bill Castle, and I'd like to take part in this discussion." I was, of course, very embarrassed; but not Castle. He was too secure in his good sense to be annoyed by criticism. We agreed that I knew more about this particular problem than he did. Castle was always willing to look at any clinical problem, and he never felt uneasy if he did not have much specific knowledge about the problem. He could identify the problem and the points at issue. He then extracted from his colleagues what they knew and added any information that he had. Knowing the general state of knowledge and the techniques available to investigators, Castle could make a reasonable guess about the knowledge that could be obtained from the library, and various members agreed to look up the relevant paper. Knowing the state of the art, he could project the next experimental approach to unearth new knowledge. A wise man, he had defined a clinical problem, collated information from persons present at the bedside, decided on the necessary library work and projected the next clinical research on the problem—all without a complete and comprehensive knowledge of the subject. He taught me that I need not know everything to be an effective teacher. When I visit other hospitals, the resident is frequently surprised that I will see any type of patient in front of a large group without special preparation. The Castle approach gives me that freedom.

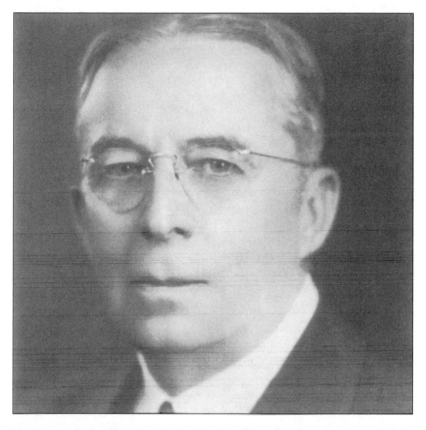

Dr. James E. Paullin, Stead's family physician and first mentor at Grady Hospital and Emory University in Atlanta.

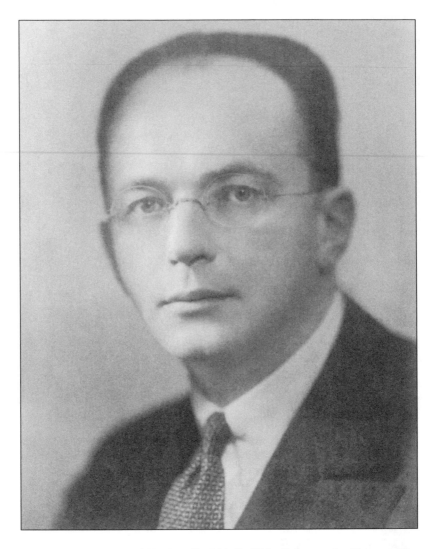

Dr. Soma Weiss in 1938, Stead's Chief of Medicine at the Boston City Hospital and the Peter Bent Brigham Hospital in Boston. Weiss died suddenly in 1942 of a subarachnoid hemorrhage.

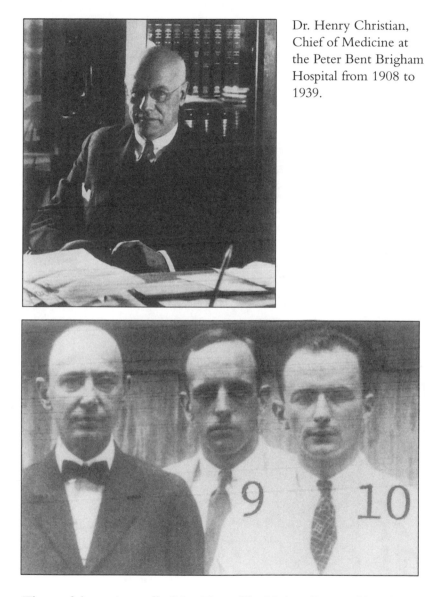

Dr. Henry Christian, Chief of Medicine at the Peter Bent Brigham Hospital from 1908 to 1939.

Three of the senior staff of the Thorndike Unit at Boston City Hospital that influenced Eugene Stead: George Minot (left), William Castle (middle), and Soma Weiss (right). Photograph taken in 1929.

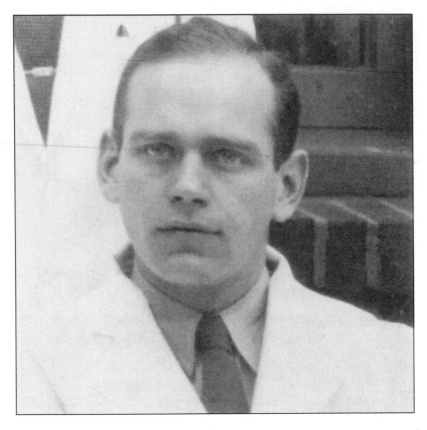

Eugene A. Stead, Jr. as a young faculty member of the Department of Medicine at the Peter Bent Brigham Hospital in Boston in 1940, age 32.

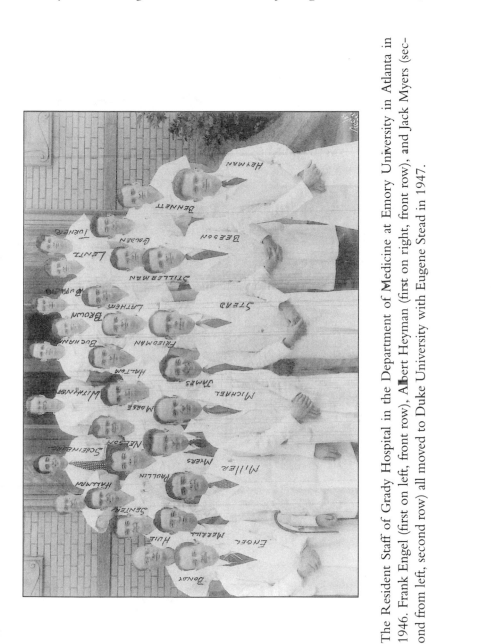

The Resident Staff of Grady Hospital in the Department of Medicine at Emory University in Atlanta in 1946. Frank Engel (first on left, front row), Albert Heyman (first on right, front row), and Jack Myers (second from left, second row) all moved to Duke University with Eugene Stead in 1947.

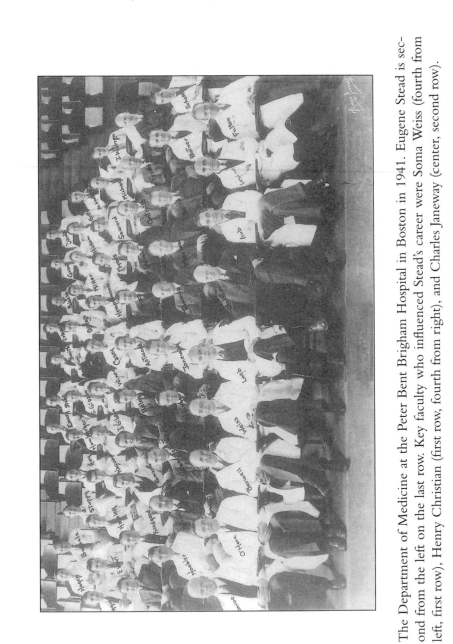

The Department of Medicine at the Peter Bent Brigham Hospital in Boston in 1941. Eugene Stead is second from the left on the last row. Key faculty who influenced Stead's career were Soma Weiss (fourth from left, first row), Henry Christian (first row, fourth from right), and Charles Janeway (center, second row).

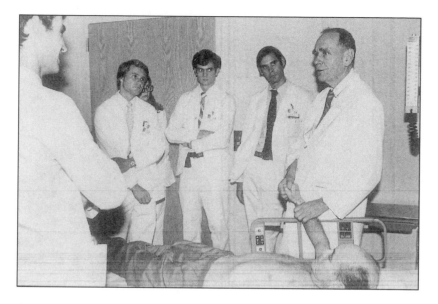

Eugene A Stead, Jr. teaching Duke Medicine housestaff at the bedside. Stead's rounds were informative, exciting, sometimes intimidating, but always held with the patient, not the disease, as the focus of the discussion.

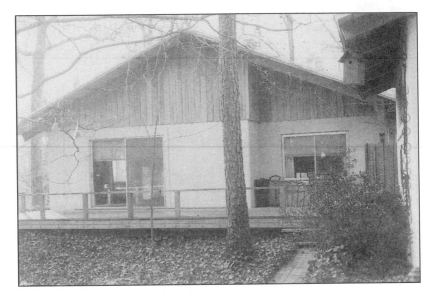

The House that the Stead Family Built. Although a work-oriented academic physician, administrator, and scientist, Eugene Stead saved ample time for his family. He did this by renting a house on the Duke University campus while he was on the faculty, and on weekends his family went to Bullock, North Carolina, 45 miles from Durham, and together built this home on Kerr Lake near the North Carolina-Virginia border. All of the Stead children now have their own homes and families, and Eugene and Evelyn Stead continue to live in the "house that the Steads built."

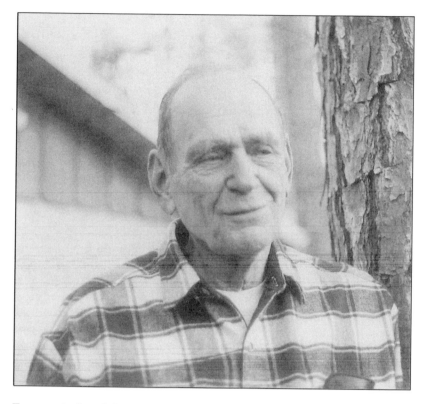

Eugene A. Stead, Jr. in 1995 at the age of 86.

III

Doctors and Patients

*T*act, sympathy and understanding are expected of the physician, for the patient is no mere collection of symptoms, signs, disordered functions, damaged organs and disturbed emotions. The patient is human, fearful and hopeful, seeking relief, help and reassurance. To the physician, as to the anthropologist, nothing human is strange or repulsive.

Chapter 14 ☞

Good Will toward Men

C hristmas is coming and our thoughts turn toward ways of making this a better world. None of us knows how to bring about "peace on earth" but each of us can contribute to the ideal of "good will toward men." Family doctors, by the breadth of their experience and by their dealing with life in all its phases and the death which comes to each of us, have the best opportunity to develop the deep understanding of human behavior and tolerance of biologic phenomena which truly allow them to manifest "good will toward men."

There are people who make significant contributions to society and others who are destructive to society. The fortunate folk who perform well tend to take personal credit for their fine performance and to look with some disdain on those who perform less well. In reality the good performers are due no personal credit. Their DNA and favorable environmental forces have molded a machine which functions well to meet the needs of the current society. Make the necessary changes in their nervous and endocrine systems and they will quickly become useless to society, and no amount of "will-power" will counteract the structural change. People disdained by society are also physical machines whose structure has been deter-mined by the interaction of their DNA and their environment. They will remain useless unless some change in structure occurs. They are not bad people. They merely represent poorly built machines.

If one wishes to change the behavior of people, one must change the anatomy of their nervous systems. Purposeful modification of human DNA will not occur for many years. Favorable changes in the next generation must come from modifications of structure produced by manipulation of the environment. Better nutrition of parents, prevention of infections and biochemical changes unfavorable to the foetus, better nutrition and living conditions for infants and children, and improved techniques for training and educating the young so that patterns useful for both intellectual and social purposes will be formed in the central nervous system, offer us our best chance to mold the anatomy of the nervous system of our future generations.

Will many of our yet-to-be-born children lack the optimal chance for favorable development? Will lack of proper nutrition and health and lack of properly timed stimuli to mold the nervous system hamper the growth of many children? We know that unfortunately the answer is "yes!" All of us would like to change that answer. The question is how. Let the spirit of Christmas inspire in each of us our own best answer.

Chapter 15 ☞

Pay the Bill Cheerfully

*T*he biologic potentialities of man are determined by the arrangements of the purine and pyrimidine bases in the chromosomes of the cell resulting from the union of the egg and sperm. The degree to which these biologic potentials are realized are a function of the environment. A knowledge of the interplay between these two forces that determine the structure and function of mankind is of obvious importance to the physician.

For the physician, modern genetics highlight the fact that every organism is an individual with its own biological potential. The role of physicians is to identify these individual characteristics and to modify the environment in such a way that the desirable potentials are fully developed and the undesirable potentials minimized. Physicians know that, from the beginning, every organism is different and that this difference will be accentuated by environmental factors.

This concept is, of course, familiar to us all. An oak tree on the rocky shores of the Pacific Coast beaten by the full force of the wind may be small and gnarled, yet its acorns will grow a stately oak in a more favorable environment.

As the years have gone by, we have realized how much the genetic possibilities can remain masked in the absence of the proper environmental stimulus. The child with galactosemia will thrive normally if milk is avoided. The middle-aged man will not develop diabetes if his weight is controlled. The primaquine-sensitive person will not develop anemia if he does not come in contact with the drug; the susceptible infant will not develop goiter if soybean milk is not used.

In clinical medicine we try to identify how the particular organism (our patient) differs from all other persons. We try to identify the factors that limit his performance. We try to find the peculiarities that make one type of living more desirable for him than others. In general, we go about this in the following way:

1. We take a family history that helps identify some of the genetic peculiarities of the patient and the effects of certain types of environmental stress on this type of genetic structure.

2. We carry out a physical examination to determine in what ways the patient differs from the average person.

3. We measure a number of physiologic and biochemical functions, again in an attempt to find out how the patient differs from others.

4. We listen to our patient's account of the effects of stress, physical and emotional, on the ability of his body to function normally. From the history alone we may define the fact that our patient does well in certain situations and does poorly in others. We do not have to understand the reasons for each of these peculiarities to put this information to therapeutic use. All of us can tell whether a car will start on a cold day even though we have little knowledge of the actual working of the automobile.

Our therapeutic approach is based on the following considerations:

1. Since all the machines are made differently and since each has been modified in different ways by the wear of life, they do not have equal capacities or equal uses. If we can determine the situations under which the organism functions best, we can make its performance improve. No worker in the laboratory

would attempt to measure infrared rays with an instrument sensitive only to the ultraviolet. Just as each laboratory instrument has its limitations, so does each organism.

2. Knowing that the machine has limitations in areas of physical performance, intellectual work, and in emotional adjustments to complex situations, and that these limitations are permanent and are characteristic of the person, we are willing to accept the limitations and not expect of the patient performances that are clearly impossible for him. Every wife discovers that her husband behaves in certain ways that seem irrational to her, but which are part of him and are not susceptible to change. The husband learns the same thing about his wife.

We are not free to do everything. The bonds of heredity and the grooves worked by environment allow little play, and the behavior of man is remarkably repetitious. Knowledge that these limitations are not self-imposed but are a reflection of the overall biological processes present allow us to be patient with persons who present us with problems that are difficult to solve. This reflection helps us to recognize that care of particular patients may be either easy or difficult, but that patients cannot be divided into good patients and bad patients.

3. Having identified the areas where the patient breaks down under stress, we can do the following:

a. Strengthen the part, if possible, by improving mechanical parts or by adding material that is lacking.

b. Avoid the stress. What is stress for the particular patient has to be learned by observation.

c. If we elect not to avoid the stress and protect a weak area, then we should pay the bill cheerfully.

Chapter 16 ☞

Brain Sorting

E ach disease resides in a person, and that person's behavior and perception of the world are functions of the structure of his unique brain. Just as diseases can be sorted and placed in categories, the brains of the persons with the diseases can be sorted. We sort the diseases by placing like with like, and brains can be sorted in the same manner. Doctors usually do not sort brains. They appreciate that we do not know the intimate architecture of the black box (brain). Not knowing the details of structure, they make no attempt to place like with like. They forget that diseases were categorized and sorted into boxes long before we understood the anatomy of the illness. The purpose of this essay is to stimulate doctors to become more active sorters of brains, and in this way to enjoy more fully the wonderful diversity of the people they care for who happen to have disease.

Neurologists sort brains of their patients when changes of structure which produce major defects in motor, sensory or autonomic functions have occurred. I, on the other hand, am interested in the sorting of brains when the neurologist reports a normal neurological examination.

Structure Determines Function and Changes in Structure Are Heralded by Changes in Function

Doctors continually care for diseases that occur in people.

They learn by experience to become expert in caring for these diseases. They effectively sort the diseases into various categories and they know that each disease state is accompanied by anatomical changes which produce changes in function which we equate with illness.

Our concept of structure (anatomy) has changed over the years. At one time we recognized only those structural changes which were visible to our unaided eye. Then we appreciated changes detectable with the light microscope. In more recent years, electron microscopy, fluorescent microscopy, isotopic labeling, and labeling with antibodies and antigens have allowed us to detect structural changes of small dimensions. We know that drugs and hormones produce changes in function because they alter the structures of membranes, enzymes, proteins, lipids or nuclei.

In the majority of instances we have detected differences in the function of a system before the anatomical changes responsible for the altered function were defined. Because of the presence of the menstrual cycle, we knew that cyclic changes in structure occurred each month long before the hypothalamic, pituitary, ovarian, uterine axis was understood in terms of hormones.

In other organs, tissues, and cells we have observed differences in function long before we have determined the anatomical changes responsible for the differences. We have accepted without question the fact that eventually the structural differences made known by the observed functional differences would be defined. Dr. James Herrick years ago observed that the red cells in a hereditary anemia found in blacks distorted light passing through a microscope in a manner different from the red cells of non-anemic white persons. He had discovered sickle cell anemia. For many years sickle cell anemia was defined solely by this abnormal distortion of the path of light. Conceptually everyone knew that the sickled cell had a structure that differed from a non-sickled normal cell and that eventually this difference in structure would be defined. Progress was slow because the persons observing the sickling were medical doctors unskilled in relating large changes in function to small changes in structure. A chance conversation between two distinguished investigators from different disciplines—William Castle, the Harvard clinical investigator, and Linus Pauling, the chemist expert in defining molecular structure—led to the observation that electrophoresis could separate sickle cell hemoglobin from normal hemoglobin because of differences in electric charge. It was a number of years later before the precise change in an amino acid responsible for the difference in charge was defined.

In the beginning, we regarded structure as relatively fixed and considered reversible changes as functional rather than structural. In reality, the change in structure preceded the change in function. Oxyhemoglobin has a different structure than reduced hemoglobin. Oxyhemoglobin has the ability to dissociate oxygen below a certain pressure. Reduced hemoglobin has the ability to attach oxygen at certain pressures of oxygen. The fact that structural differences were present was first defined by these reactions to oxygen and not by analysis of the two hemoglobins by x-ray crystallography. We knew that there had to be two different structures because identical structures behave in the same way and non-identical structures behave in different ways.

To predict differences in function by determining differences in structure requires a much more advanced state of knowledge. Even when we can define the difference in structure precisely, as in sickle cell hemoglobin, we still use as our first screening maneuver the functional test defining the differences in response of the abnormal red cells to light. In 1942, clinicians knew that the kidney frequently ceased functioning in the presence of shock and infection. The pathologist of that era was unable to define an anatomical change responsible for the renal failure. The lack of structural definition caused no harm because the clinician knew that changes in the kidney as yet unrecognized by the pathologist had produced the anuria. During World War II the pathologic changes were defined, and the condition of acute tubular necrosis was recognized.

Structure and Function in the Brain

It is worth pausing to consider the progress that has been made in complex biologic situations where differences in behavior were known to exist but it seemed unlikely that the anatomical arrangements responsible for the behavior would ever be determined. In my medical school days, proteins were mysterious and what little was known about them had no medical application. Chromosomes were known to be related to heredity but the possibility that we could understand the molecular basis for heredity was perceived only dimly. The importance of the immune system was appreciated, but the means to investigate this system and turn it into a medical discipline were lacking. Some proteins were known to function as enzymes but their structure was not defined. At that time, leaders in medicine could properly say that doctors should not concern themselves about proteins, heredity, enzymes, and immunology because patients could not be helped by knowledge in these areas. Doctors were advised to spend their time in areas where their activities relieved pain, prevented disability, and postponed death by the application of the scientific method to patients.

Today some of our medical leaders tell us that human behavior is not a problem relevant to medicine and should be ignored by doctors who instead should concentrate on the relief of pain, the prevention of suffering, and the postponement of death by the application of scientific principles.

The fact that differences in function define differences in structure is accepted and used by all students of medicine for all organs except the brain. The complexity of human behavior, the complexity of the structural organization of the brain, and the acceptance of the spirit and mind as attributes separate from the structure of the brain have all tended to obscure the obvious— namely, that at any one point in time the response of the brain to inputs is determined by its structure. By observing the response to multiple inputs, brains can be sorted into a series of boxes, each box containing brains structurally more similar than those in the other boxes.

Resistance to the Concept That Structure of the Brain Determines Behavior

Why has the study of the brain and behavior not been more eagerly pursued by most doctors? Most doctors have not accepted the fact that behavior is a function of the structure of the brain and that the structure of an individual brain will eventually be determined. Behavior is still thought of in mystical terms. The second reason for physician resistance is that one has to deal with each brain as an important entity whose structure can be altered by a nearly infinite number of inputs, both within and without the body. A large part of the structure of the brain is genetically determined, but environment and use of the system can greatly modify the mature system. The science of immunology deals with averages. One aberrant lymphocyte may evolve into cancer and destroy the body, but one aberrant brain can detonate an atom bomb and obliterate New York City. Because of the nearly infinite variations in brains and the importance of a single brain, classifications are more complex than those customarily handled by biologists. We are afraid of learning too much about the brain. Each of us has his own ideas about what is good and bad. If we understand the structure of the brain and can alter its development and structure by manipulation, we can change human behavior. We are willing to have the brain altered by mixing gene pools, by intrauterine influences and by the effects of culture, education, poverty, and drugs as long as these operate in a random and unstructured way. Definitive control of brain structure frightens us. Doctors in the past have offered too much and accomplished too little. The fundamental characteristics of an individual adult brain can be altered very little by verbal inputs from doctors and other people. By observing the outputs from brains, one can appreciate the complexity of the structure and the degree of uniqueness. Knowing that two brains are different poses a problem in biology. The problem is to define the differences in molecular and cellular terms. The appreciation of the fact that there is an interesting biologic and biomedical problem does not translate into immediately useful therapy.

Psychoanalysis has performed a great service by demonstrating that the structure of the adult brain is the sum of genetic and environmental influences that begin *in utero* and have their greatest effect in infancy and childhood. Once the structure is set, analytic techniques are useful in defining differences and serve as a useful input for sorting brains. The analysts have also shown how difficult it is to change the structure of the adult brain by talking.

The thesis of this paper is that doctors who know that behavior is a function of the brain can, by observing behavior, sort brains into a number of useful categories using the same methodology that allows us to sort diseases involving different structures in the body into medically useful categories. The appreciation that similarities and differences in the structure of brains can be determined by noninvasive testing opens up wide areas where the doctor can be useful.

Plasticity of the Brain

The brain in the embryo is relatively plastic, and its structure, developing in accordance with its genetic code, is capable of major modifications from environmental influences. For a time the baby *in utero* was thought to be well protected from environmental influences. Erythroblastosis fetalis, the tragedy of thalidomide, the effects of thyroid dysfunction and hyperinsulinism on the newborn baby, the deformities induced by rubella virus, the small babies of malnourished mothers, and the large babies of diabetic mothers demonstrate the fallacy of assuming that environmental influences cannot cause major changes in the fetus.

A number of years ago we were confident that we could separate environmental and genetic mechanisms for change. The knowledge that viruses can become incorporated into genes, and that this new genetic material can be transmitted by chromosomes has made the separation between environmental and genetic mechanisms less certain.

The brain at birth is one-half adult size; 74% of adult size at 18 months of age; 90% at four years. During childhood the brain reaches adult size. By birth, there is some evidence of myelinization in most parts of the central nervous system. The peak period of myelinization occurs postnatally after the peak activity of glial formation. Some glial cells form during fetal life, but their chief proliferation occurs in the early months after birth. Dendritic elaboration occurs actively at the same time.

The brain as it ages becomes less and less plastic. The child developing in a home where French, English, and German are routinely spoken has no difficulty in conversing with each of the family members in their native tongue. The ability of a child to speak in several languages with little effort is lost before the average child is exposed to a foreign language. Possession of absolute pitch is related to the age at which training on a musical instrument is begun. Of those who begin training before the age of four years, 95% possess absolute pitch compared to only 3% of those who start training between 12 and 14 years.

In a child, a major lesion of the speech areas of the left hemisphere produces transfer of the whole speech mechanism to the right hemisphere. Thus the usually speechless right hemisphere can under certain conditions become a language hemisphere, just like the left.

The effect of disuse on the structure of the plastic nervous system of the child is illustrated by loss of vision which occurs when muscle imbalance causes enough diplopia to require the suppression of the image from one eye. In a surprisingly short time, atrophic changes occur in the connections to the suppressed eye and loss of function occurs because of permanent changes in neurons of the primary visual cortex. All data indicate that the general pattern of the visual system is genetically determined, but the subtle details of morphology and function are modifiable through visual experience at least during the first few years of life.

Thus, the brain as it develops can change its structure by environmental inputs. It can lose substance by non-use. It can permanently facilitate connections by inputs which form habit patterns. At the same time, structural changes in the brain are occurring as the body makes and distributes chemicals which attach to receptors in the central nervous system. The degree of changeability that the locus of cortical functions can undergo is different for different functions.

Reversible and Irreversible Changes in Structure of the Brain

Mothers and fathers produce changes in the structure of the nervous system of their children by training and education.

Habits result from repetitive inputs into the nervous system. The first time around, the change induced is easily reversible and the brain may revert to its original state. By the time toilet training is completed, the repetition has produced permanent structural changes which will stay in place until degenerative or disease states change the structure of the brain where the habit was imprinted.

The adult brain is composed of (1) structures that are fixed and unchangeable except by aging and disease, (2) structures that can be changed reversibly by the expenditure of large amounts of energy, and (3) structures that are easily reversible. Because of the continual change in the reversible portion of the structure, one has to be reminded that behavior at any one point in time is a function of the structure of the brain at that point in time. Reversible changes in structure occur with learning, thinking, sleeping, and waking. The majority of drugs, hormones, and neurotransmitters cause reversible changes in structure which can be defined by functional testing.

By the time one enters medical school, the brain has many parts where the structural changes induced by genes and environment are irreversible, or reversible only with a great expenditure of energy. This is very obvious in the part of the brain that determines the feeling state. I have not found laboratory experiments to confirm or negate my clinical impressions that the portions of the brain determining attitudes and feeling states become less plastic at an earlier date than the portions of the brain tested by standardized college board examination. Attitudes toward parents, peers, authority figures, religious beliefs, fantasies, fears, happiness, sexuality, and a variety of habits good and bad are firmly fixed in structure at an early date. In our naïveté, many of us have presumed that religious wars had yielded to reason. Ayotollah Khomeini, the Irish, the Jews and Arabs have reminded us that religious wars are a reality and that brain changing is difficult.

The portions of our brains concerned with memory and the qualities tested by our college and medical school aptitude and achievement tests retain a greater degree of plasticity. All education and training is based on the fact that structural changes are still possible. Observation makes me believe that by the time a student enters medical school, the irreversible portions of the structure of the brain have become so dominant that the top ceiling for performance has been set. Environmental and educational stimuli will determine the degree to which one climbs toward that ceiling.

Brain Sorting

I was fortunate in having a clinical and laboratory apprenticeship under Soma Weiss,[1] one of the great clinicians of the 1930s. He was aware of the importance of the nervous system in regulating and modifying the behavior of the heart and circulatory system.

From that time on, I have been interested in what I call brain sorting: putting like brains into the same basket. Since the brains I dealt with were in live persons I could not use anatomical techniques, but I knew that the brains with identical responses to a wide variety of inputs would be similar in structure and that brains with a great divergence in outputs from my battery of inputs would be different. I could therefore sort brains into subgroups without knowing the precise anatomical configurations underlying the subgroups.

My first observations were on myself. I had discovered early that I was tune deaf. On the day of the 1981 Kentucky Derby, I heard the announcer state that the band always plays "My Old

---

1. See Chapter 11.

Kentucky Home" on Derby Day. When the music struck up, I told my wife that my ability to recognize tunes had improved: I knew the band was playing "My Old Kentucky Home"! She rejoined that everyone was rising to their feet and that the band was playing "The Star Spangled Banner." I also have a relative deficit in recognizing form and shape. I cannot draw my wife's face. I have never known the color of anyone's eyes. I did know that color blindness could be easily determined and that this disorder had to have an as yet undetermined anatomical basis.

Georgia O'Keeffe says, "The meaning of a word—to me—is not as exact as the meaning of a color. Color and shapes make a more definite statement than words." By contrast, when Gene Stead says a word, he forms a picture in his brain that is much more specific and concrete than the image imprinted on his brain when he sees a picture of the scene described by the word.

The parents of a child with dyslexia or stuttering have had a great burden lifted from them with the knowledge that these difficulties have an anatomical basis and are not caused by interpersonal relationships. Children who learn slowly in social situations do so because the inputs that create usual pictures in most people create different images in the brain of the slow social learner. These persons can be helped by teaching them to find out what the more average person has seen and then to correct their own pictures. That the neurological disability remains is easily demonstrable when a new situation is created and the old cues used to revise the pictures are not applicable.

Can knowledge that behavior is determined by the structure of the brain and that the brains with different structures can be grouped together be useful in the practice of medicine? I think that it can be useful. I'm in the minority because few generalists or specialists are interested in brain sorting.

The knowledge that the structure of the brain puts a top level on performance is the basis of tolerance of one human for another. It highlights the importance of selecting brains that can perform the functions that are expected of them and the necessity of accepting the fact that each brain has some structural limitations and cannot give an equally high level of output in all areas.

For many years I offered my chief residents the opportunity of working with a distinguished Chinese psychoanalyst, Bingham Dai.[2] I had been impressed by the repetitive reactions of these talented young physicians. In person-to-person reactions, they behaved predictably, wasted a large amount of energy, became fatigued and, as far as I could see, learned nothing about themselves or the persons with whom they were reacting. Working with Dr. Dai, they came to accept their uniqueness. They realized that they were excellent in many areas but limited in others. They discovered that their brains limited their behavior and that brain changing was difficult.

Ability to make high grades in school and excel in aptitude tests may not translate into an outstanding performance in our irrationally-run world. Performance is greatly modified by the non-IQ portions of our brains. The more persons touched in the course of the day the more limiting becomes the non-IQ portion of the brain. I am performance-sensitive and examination-insensitive. To belong to my team, one's assets must exceed his liabilities. We arrange your work to make the greatest use of your assets and to minimize your liabilities. We will not attempt to change you. The general frame of reference for most people is that a person can achieve any goal that they desire. My own frame of reference is that people are limited by the structure of their brains and that no one person can be all things to all people.

Again, we go back to biologic diversity. Within the area of

2. Bingham Dai was a Ph.D. psychologist in the Department of Psychiatry, Duke University Medical Center.

our so-called normal, there are wide ranges of function. A person with normal muscular coordination may not have the coordination to be an outstanding athlete; a person with normal sight may not see in a flower the pictures that form in the brain of Georgia O'Keeffe; a person with normal hearing may be tone deaf; a person with a high IQ may be dyslexic; a person with great artistic ability is often intolerant of lesser artists; a great scholar may always be stubbing his toe in a variety of social settings; prejudice against women or blacks may color the view of a politician; various blank areas such as color blindness, lack of sense of direction or shape appreciation may be present. A person may have structural changes which cause short attention span, low opinion of himself, envy, fear, sexual dysfunction, and a variety of other manifestations. Certain structures and their corresponding functions may not be completely absent but there may be enough alteration to markedly modify the fit between man and his environment. The majority of identifiable differences in brain structure demonstrated by the functional differences described above are overlooked in the usual medical examination. Yet these differences in structure of the brain become very significant when one observes how patients with different brains relate to their environment.

People with diseases have all the problems of well persons, plus the problems created by illness. Given the choice, I have preferred to care for well persons with symptoms rather than for persons being consumed by destructive illness. My preferred population is more flexible and the potential performance is higher. Most of my colleagues prefer to treat persons with more severe illness because the illness so dominates the picture that they can ignore the differences in brain structure and function that I find so fascinating.

Advantages Accruing to the Doctor who Knows That the Structure of the Brain Determines Behavior

Do doctors who know that behavior is determined by the structure of the brain and who have developed an ability to determine differences in brains by observing behavior practice medicine differently from doctors who do not have this approach to practice? I believe they do, and I will detail some of the differences.

1. Doctors are tolerant of the behavior of their patients, of their colleagues, and of their families. They are aware that their behavior is a function of their unique brain structure, and they know that they cannot be all things to all people. Their patients and colleagues must accept them as they are. To change their behavior they must change their brain. Knowing that the behavior of their patients is a brain function, and that patients have only a limited ability to change the brain, doctors will accept patients as they are and not require them to conform to doctors' norms of behavior. They will comfortably care for the complaining portion of the population who have healthy bodies that are poorly used without a feeling of superiority.

2. Doctors will build a stronger office and hospital support team because they will select persons whose brains can meet the demands of their practice. They will know that each person brings assets and liabilities. They will not retain anyone whose liabilities exceed their assets. They will not be disappointed when the patterns of behavior brought to the practice persist.

3. Doctors will enjoy their spouses and children because they will accept the individuality of family members and not require that they be like them.

4. In interviews with patients, doctors will look for the wear and tear caused by poor brain-environment interactions. They

will identify the assets and liabilities of their patients and help them appreciate their own uniqueness. Once this uniqueness is accepted, they can help devise ways to use their assets and minimize their liabilities.

5. If doctors are teachers, they will identify the differences among their students. They will help each student develop his or her own form of excellence, and will not require that students adapt to their own excellence.

6. Knowing that function is a manifestation of structure, doctors will drop the distinction between functional and organic illness. All complaining comes from the brain. The structure of the brain and inputs to it from peripheral organs and the environment determine the pattern of the complaining.

7. Doctors who know that the structure of the brain determines behavior will make the distinction between pain that is commonly caused by a massive inflow of impulses from the periphery and suffering that is a function of the higher regions of the brain and can occur with little or no input from peripheral organs. They will know that pain predominates in acute situations but that suffering becomes more of a problem in chronic situations. The distinction between pain and suffering is very important when the presence of pain signals to the patient the threat of death.

I recently saw a 58 year-old man on his third admission to Duke Medical Center for intractable angina pectoris. The doctor in charge knew little about the patient's educational background, religious beliefs, hopes, aspirations, and fears. He also did not know the changes in the brain produced by the education that the patient had received from his contacts with doctors and nurses. The belief systems of the wife and family and the effect of the illness on their behavior were unknown by the doctor.

The patient had a two-hour episode of pain of moderate severity seven days before he was first seen in the Duke ambulatory clinic. The doctor correctly suspected coronary disease and obtained an electrocardiogram which showed the findings of a recent myocardial infarct. The patient was placed on a stretcher and rushed to the coronary care unit. A more thoughtful doctor, knowing about doctor-induced changes in the brain and the likelihood of starting a pattern of suffering, would have been much more relaxed. In the absence of arrhythmia and any signs of congestive failure, home care would have been more appropriate for this 7-day old infarct.

The New York Heart Association's division of patients with angina pectoris into four classes is not helpful in evaluating treatment because one never knows whether the disability is caused by pain or by suffering. Cardiologists need to look beyond the heart in evaluating the outcomes of various forms of therapy.

8. Doctors knowing that behavior is a manifestation of the structure of the brain appreciate that even minimal brain changing requires time and energy. They will determine the one or two changes that they wish to make and structure their care of the patient to accomplish this limited goal. If diet is of overwhelming importance, they will not diffuse their efforts by adding drugs. If stopping smoking is the key to alleviating bronchitis and asthma, they will put a major amount of effort into the venture. If early ambulation is the primary postoperative goal, doctors will be sparing in medication and generous in their praise to the patient, to the nurses, and to the family on every trip around the unit. The most common mistake in medical practice is to not appreciate the effort required for brain change. Too much is asked of the patient with too little expenditure of energy by doctors. Doctors forget that to change behavior they must change the brain.

9. Doctors aware of the plasticity of the brain *in utero* and early childhood will be more active in devising social systems that realize that the brains of young children are our most

important resource. It may or may not be desirable to give economic bonuses for having more children. It is certainly desirable to provide adequate support—financial and emotional—to any children who are brought into this world. The doctor knowledgeable about the structural basis of behavior will know that the care of well children is more important than the care of any other dependent group.

The doctor aware of the fact that behavior is a function of the brain will have a different attitude toward members of our society who have had their brains changed by poorly designed social legislation. The average doctor is angry when he finds veterans, welfare clients, and various forms of double-dippers milking the system for undeserved benefits. Society has established laws that modify brains in unfavorable ways. The doctor needs to educate lawmakers about the basis of human behavior and help them to avoid traps which have made much of our social legislation fail to accomplish what we intended. The responsibility for the changed brain which produces the behavior which outrages the doctor can be charged more properly to society than to the individual.

Who Should Teach Human Behavior?

Students need to understand the structure of the brain—gross, microscopic and submicroscopic—and the outputs from this complex structure that we call behavior. They need to know that to change behavior, they must alter the structure of the brain. They need to appreciate that many structural differences are called to our attention by observing that a particular brain functions in a different way from other brains. Whether one can define the precise change in structure producing the observed differences in function is a function of the state of the anatomical and pathological arts.

Behavior should be taught by the portion of the faculty that can keep the obligatory relationship between structure and function in sharp focus at all times. It should not be taught by anyone who talks about "functional illness" or by any group who in describing the outputs of the brain lists neurologic findings in one column and psychologic findings in another column. It should not be taught by the neurologist who when asked to see a patient with chronic pancreatitis who is pain-free but refuses to ingest food says, "Don't call me; it's not a neurologic problem." At the preclinical level, human behavior should be taught by the faculty who traditionally relate structure to function. These persons are usually found in the departments of Anatomy, Physiology, Pharmacology, and Pathology.

At the clinical level, behavior is best taught by doctors who care for patients who are going to live productively for years but who are limited in part by brain-environment interaction problems. These doctors need to know how to define structural changes by functional testing and to be able to sort brains into useful groups.

The Doubting Thomases

My more sophisticated colleagues will ask: what's the fuss? Everyone knows that behavior results from the structure of the brain. During professional life, I have examined patients with students at all levels. I have asked these students many questions. I know that they have a mystical frame of reference for human behavior and that this frame is very different from that which they use to learn about the heart or kidney. They always attempt to distinguish between functional and organic illness. They are unable to define functional illness in useful terms. They learn little from practice about the people who have the diseases. If each of my critics will observe himself and his speech carefully, he will be surprised how often he slips up and forgets that structure determines function and that a change in function requires a change in structure. I quote a distinguished neurologist, Mac-Donald Critchley: "Is this a psychiatric affection, that is to say one which is psychologically determined? I submit that it is not; but it is an organic affection of obscure origin." Critchley has figured out that functional testing allows us to recognize some as yet undetermined changes in structure of the brain, but he still is not convinced in his heart of hearts that all human behavior is determined by the structure of the brain.

Chapter 17 ☞

Doctoring Is Difficult

A patient comes to a doctor with a complaint. The first problem doctors must solve is complex—is this patient ill or well?

The patient's complaint may arise because

(a) a well body is equipped with a sensitive nervous system that detects changes induced by the environment that are not detected by less sensitive systems; or

(b) a well body is being used in a way that will make most bodies complain; or

(c) the patient's nondiseased but nevertheless highly individualized body is being used in a way that would not make most well bodies complain, but does make his well—though somewhat different—body complain; or

(d) illness is raising its ugly head.

To determine the origin of the complaint and to judge whether it represents illness requires the doctor to define health and illness. A little reflection will show that these definitions are not easy. Two years ago I gave a medical student this task. We have since avoided further discussion of his assignment, because he has not written any simple definitions of health and illness, and I have not been able to help him. We cannot define health by any particular level of performance. The person with the highest I.Q. is not healthier than the person with an average I.Q.

The person who can run 100 yards in 10 seconds is not necessarily healthier than one of his or her slower compatriots. Is the person born with one leg missing diseased? He or she is certainly a person who can be helped by the medical profession.

In general, we believe that persons who show no signs of change but exhibit different performance levels are not ill but are examples of the fact that each person is put together differently. We do not expect a tractor to be interchangeable with a Rolls Royce, and if we try to get the same performance out of the tractor and the Rolls Royce, we will be in serious trouble.

The patient comes to the doctor complaining of many things. He may or may not have a disease. If the body is healthy but poorly used, the role of the doctor is to recognize the absence of illness and to make a better fit between the patient and his environment. The patient will be much better able to cope with the problem if he realizes that well bodies poorly used may result in much discomfort and complaining. If illness is present, that fact must be faced by both doctor and patient.

The patient going to the doctor with complaints commonly assumes that he is ill. If doctors prescribe medication or other therapy without carefully distinguishing—to the patient as well as to themselves—when they are caring for a patient as a healthy person with complaints and when they are treating illness, the patient's assumption of illness is reinforced. The reality of the complaining is not the point at issue. The question is, Is illness the cause of the complaining?

The fact that this question is not easy to answer simply means doctoring is difficult.

Chapter 18

Traps and Stratagems of Diagnosis

*T*he diagnostic procedure is a fascinating exercise. It involves the most acute use of our senses and the accurate recording of our observations. Doctors must synthesize in their central nervous systems information from the patient and his family, from other doctors who have cared for the patient in the past, from colleagues in various specialties who are helping with the immediate problem, and from laboratory data. Prognosis and correct therapy depend upon the correct use of the diagnostic process.

A diagnosis written in a record has an entirely different meaning. It consists of a single word or a few phrases. The person reading the diagnosis is supposed to be able to create in his mind's eye the entire clinical picture. The written diagnosis is the shorthand summary of the complete diagnostic procedure.

The diagnosis, as entered in the record, leaves out much of the information normally available during the diagnostic process. The assumption is made that all of the data have been collected accurately and interpreted correctly. The noise that appears in all communications systems and is inevitable when data are collected from multiple sources and persons of different competency is disregarded.

The doctor in training will state that the patient was treated for an acute myocardial infarction three months ago. The doctor with experience will always ask: "The diagnosis was supported by what data?" He is interested in the setting of the illness, the experiences of the patient, the behavior of the doctor and the objective evidence to support the conclusion that some heart muscle died. The young doctor wants to conserve time by accepting the diagnosis of myocardial infarction. The older doctor wants to accumulate all available information and maintain as many options as possible. The young doctor can transmit his information in three words—acute myocardial infarction—but his chance of error-making is far greater.

This problem of evaluating information and using it intelligently is common in any communication system. An object is spotted in the sky. It is identified correctly or incorrectly as a hostile airplane (in our hypothetical patient—myocardial infarction). There is no difficulty in the transfer of information and the object is promptly shot down. If identification is deferred and all choices remain open, a tremendous amount of information must be continually transmitted and wide bands for communication must be available. The chance of a friendly airplane (or a significant medical finding) being destroyed because of error in identification is greatly increased. When the choice is narrowed, the information is easy to transmit but the opportunity for error-making is increased. When all the information is transferred, the equipment required is complex, the dollar cost is high, but error is reduced.

The transfer of information by the use of diagnostic terms is convenient shorthand and effective when medicine is simple. When medicine is hard, a review of the diagnostic procedures must replace the acceptance of the diagnosis.

Chapter 19 ☙

Doctors of Experience

*E*xperienced doctors have firmly fixed in their mind a series of patterns which covers all common illnesses. They quickly identify which pattern to call up; as data from history, physical examination, laboratory/special examinations come in, they check off each item. When data fit the pattern, they do not have to pinpoint the precise numbers on their brain. They know the age of the patient by decades and round off data to fit the expected range. The blood pressure is 130/90 not 128/88. They doze away until something is found that doesn't fit the learned pattern, then they are wide awake. Does the unexpected finding mean that they have selected the wrong pattern, is it an erroneous finding to be disregarded, or is it an example of a finding known to occur in this pattern but only rarely. On to the library to check out the unexpected data. Months later doctors of experience can tell you all of the details. They describe their pattern and tell you what didn't fit and why. You are amazed at their memory.

It is helpful if anyone learning medicine begins fairly early to identify how they can carry a large amount of information with so little dependence upon memory of each individual detail. Doctors only need to remember those things that did not fit the expected pattern and that made them question whether the diagnosis was correct or whether they simply had something unusual in the commonplace. This method of remembering with a minimum of investment of energy is worth learning. This is what I do, and I think it is very effective.

Chapter 20 ☞

The White Bear Syndrome

*H*ow well disciplined is your diagnostic thinking? Dr. Willis Hurst[1] has called attention to the difficulty of thinking freely after one's mind is channeled into a particular groove. As he puts it, a person put in a quiet corner and told not to think of a white bear will, in fact, think of the white bear unless he has excellent control of his thoughts. Dr. Hurst labels this "the White Bear Syndrome." He illustrates his point with examples of errors made by doctors who had their thoughts channeled away from the correct diagnosis, and did not even consider the correct diagnosis.

Doctors must keep their minds open to a wide range of possibilities. They must consider both the usual and the rare. They must be particularly careful not to overlook the treatable. They must examine the precise evidence on which each diagnosis stands. They must be ever watchful for the second disease that develops while their attention is focused on the original diagnosis.

All of us are guilty on occasion of following a single channel of thought and missing a diagnosis that could have been made by a beginner. I was on the floor when a man was admitted with

---

1. J. Willis Hurst, MD was Chief of Medicine at Emory University from 1957–1986.

the story of vomiting blood and shock. Both radial pulses were absent and the blood pressure in the arms could not be measured. This was judged to be an emergency and the diagnosis of shock from gastric hemorrhage seemed obvious. The referring physician could not remove his mind from this channel and he missed the obvious. The patient was not pale and both femoral pulses were normal. The correct diagnoses were minor blood loss and bilateral chronic occlusive disease of both subclavian arteries. There was no emergency.

Each of us needs to recycle information that has grown rusty. We need to look again, through the eyes of our colleagues, at partially remembered material. We need constant intake to move us from our prejudices and avoid the White Bear Syndrome.

Chapter 21

The Use of the Fundus to Demonstrate the Complexity of Communication

I have had a long-time interest in the examination of the fundus with the ophthalmoscope. I early learned that you can make more detailed observations through a dilated pupil than through a small pupil. Movement of the eye allows the macular and the peripheral fundus to be visualized more easily. Changes in visibility of the blood in the arteries and veins and changes in caliber of vessels are detected much more frequently if each vessel is followed from the optic disc to the periphery.

I have often used the fundus to demonstrate the difficulty in communication. A word creates in my brain a picture. I never know how the picture formed in my brain relates to that formed in another brain unless each of us can project the brain pictures so that similarities and differences can be detected by ourselves and others. The very considerable differences that can occur in the brain images of the same object are well demonstrated by asking the resident and myself to exteriorize our brain images by drawing a picture of the fundus.

I always ask the resident whether he has drawn the fundus as it is or as it is not. From experience I know that he has drawn it as it is not. After considerable effort, he can form an accurate picture of the fundus in his brain and exteriorize this picture on paper.

We know that without a large investment of time and energy two apparently normal people cannot create comparable pictures from the symbols we call words. The complexity of the brain allows a multitude of variations in structure that are not detected by the neurologist because he does not analyze brains for their ability to project comparable pictures from a multitude of symbols.

Lawyers recognize the likelihood of two persons not receiving the same picture from words. They spend their days in trying to devise language that can create only one picture. In spite of their efforts, success is rare. The problem is compounded when one tries to create the same brain picture in two persons who have different native languages.

Imperfect communication because of the assumption that words create identical pictures is present in all fields. It is particularly troublesome between doctors and patients. Doctors know the picture they want to form in the patient's brain but they frequently forget the time and effort needed to make the transfer. Unless they form the habit of having the patient in some way exteriorize his picture for observation by the doctor, confusion will abound. Accurate communication is the single most valuable asset of the skilled doctor.

Chapter 22 ☞

Two Lessons on Communication

*M*y first lesson came from my father who, on the basis of grammar school education, was supporting a wife and five children. My sister and I broke the family bank by running up bills for two acute but extended illnesses. My father wrote each creditor explaining why the check was not in the mail but outlining his plans for eventual payment. He updated his report each month. The repayment was completed over an 18-month period. During this time he maintained an A credit rating. The first thing to learn about communicating is to remember to communicate.

Patients taught me my second lesson. Never give discharge instructions on the morning of discharge from the hospital. Give them well in advance, and on the day of discharge have the patients tell you what they have learned about the illness and what you want them to carry out at home. You never know whether you have communicated until you listen to the play-back.

I have won many nickels[1] because I read more accurately than my colleagues. Knowing that accurate recall is difficult, I spend energy on the process, and where accurate recall is impor-

---

1. Eugene Stead often livened up ward rounds by making nickel bets with the housestaff about contested diagnostic or therapeutic issues.

tant I shut my eyes and repeat the essential information. I didn't win nickels because I was smarter, but knowing that the task was difficult, I worked harder.

Communicating is facilitated if we refrain from using any words that we cannot define. If the historian tells me the name of the place where the patient lives, but has no knowledge of the location and nature of the place, he puts noise, not communication, into the dialogue. If he says that the patient has a functional illness and cannot sharply define the meaning of functional all is for naught.

There are many ways to communicate. I rarely ask young colleagues to come to my office. On the way to theirs, I see many things. The hall may be dirty; a patient may receive callous treatment from the bill collector; I see a colleague who starts a productive chain of thought. My young colleagues are impressed by my interest in them, and I have the chance to watch them at their home base. They know that I regard them as important persons because I have been willing to exert myself to communicate.

In seeing patients with colleagues—students, interns, residents, fellow practitioners, nurses, physiotherapists, pharmacists—it is important to remember there is no prearranged rank. Any person may have the needed information and should be free to share it. Any of my students who aced the professor always received an A, and the opportunity to become a medical intern. I, in turn, was smarter after the exchange. I am always willing to sacrifice ego for information. In these situations communication depends on mutual trust—not on rank or compulsion.

The faculty of the medical school have always had some problem in communicating with their students. The faculty want the students to read widely, discuss freely, and know where information is stored. At the same time they insist that every area be covered in medical school and assume that no learning will occur after graduation. They set up a series of hurdles—memory-oriented examinations—and are suprised that the students spend their time memorizing facts and never explore the many opportunities for using the fabulously equipped facilities and relating to a superb group of professionals. The faculty forget "the forgetting curve." They want at all costs to make a "safe doctor." They forget that the ability to comfortably say *I don't know but if it's important I'll find out* makes a safe doctor. The student's primary goal is not to learn but to graduate from medical school. Until we give open book, open library and open computer examinations the best of students will tend to become memory grinds. Thank God, school lasts only four years!

We have not solved the problem of communication between disciplines. I once served as a biological consultant to a group of space scientists. They were engineers and physicists. They could not grasp the complexity of biological systems where all reactions have to be facilitated by enzymes that are manufactured in thousands of discrete cell factories. They never grasped that the products of all these factories would never be identical and that every biological reaction would have a broad distribution curve. When thousands of these broad curves are summed we have the diversity so characteristic of all living things.

In interdisciplinary communication much of the day is spent in defining terms so that each group can know what is meant by words and sentences. The net effect is that the initial output of a team composed of persons from diverse disciplines is less than it would be if each person stayed within the bounds of one discipline. If the team can be housed and live together, understanding and cohesion will eventually occur. You then have a superb, flexible and productive unit. Geographic proximity and time are the only solutions I have found.

Chapter 23 ☞

Patients Who Recover

I have always been interested in self-limited illnesses of unknown etiology. These illnesses have a definite time of onset, run a widely variable course and end in complete recovery. During the course of the illness the patient needs the type of protection afforded any ill patient, but when the illness is over the patient is well and requires no further protection. The fact that the illness is self-limited is frequently masked by treatment. For this reason the frequency of this syndrome in practice is hard to determine.

The quickest way to become knowledgeable in this area is to take complete health histories in a large number of patients. The periods when the patient was out of work for more than one week or when he visited a doctor more than three times in a month are recorded. In this type of survey the diagnosis is commonly not helpful because usually it is made more from desperation than from knowledge. Of much more importance is the account of what happened. How did the patient feel? What complaints were present? What did the doctor do? What special examinations were made? What treatment was instigated? What did the wife say? How did the mother and mother-in-law react? What was the pattern of recovery? What was the total cost of the illness?

Many diseases that are usually self-limited have a known etiology and well defined pathology. Infectious hepatitis is a good example. Some are of unknown etiology but have a well enough defined clinical course and pathologic findings to allow a definitive subgrouping to which a diagnostic term can be given. Infectious mononucleosis is a good example of this group. Physicians are comfortable in the treatment of these well-defined types of self-limited illness. They are less certain when the laboratory tests are normal and when the illness extends beyond a week.

Many self-limited illnesses begin with fatigue, loss of libido and evidence of either irritability or lack of inhibition in the nervous system. Because of the absence of any laboratory tests for illness, doctors frequently wonder if the patient is ill. The patient is, of course, smarter. He knows that he is ill! The patient frequently becomes desperate because he feels that if the doctor doesn't do something he will become steadily worse. Doctors with experience know that the patient was well until a given time, has been sick until the present, and will eventually be well again. They know that they must devise a way for the patient to live until recovery occurs but that this will occur without their help. The doctor's role is to support the patient, to prevent him from making unwise decisions about the future and to avoid the development of patterns of behavior that will handicap the patient when he is well.

These episodes of self-limited illness in productive persons must be separated from experiences with patients who are chronic complainers and who have a lifetime pattern of difficulty in performing. I do not know how to draw the line between some of these episodes of self-circumscribed illness and the disease syndrome that we call depression. Both occur in productive people and both end in recovery. The wide clinical spectrum of the self-circumscribed illnesses makes it very unlikely that they can have a single etiology.

Doctors who see patients in the first days and weeks of such self-limited illness have the most difficult time. They don't know whether their patient will be alive or dead four weeks later. Doctors who see patients later have a tremendous advantage. They can eliminate all diseases that would have given definitive findings in a period of time equal to that between onset and the present. Interestingly enough in the medical center, we often see the patients after recovery begins. The clinical improvement rarely goes smoothly. One or more downturns on a generally rising curve are common. Both doctor and patient become discouraged with these downswings and referral at this point is common.

Patients are frequently apologetic for using your time when they discover that they are getting well without any definitive therapy. I have always enjoyed caring for these patients. What gives a doctor any more satisfaction than a well patient? Even if God did the curing, I kept the devil away during the period of despair.

Chapter 24 ⌒

Our Probabilistic World

My generation grew up in a relatively absolute world. Things were black or white. In a more probabilistic world, the certainty of blackness or whiteness disappears to be replaced by a probability of blackness or whiteness. The awareness of a probabilistic world rather than a certain world is creating a new series of problems for those of us practicing medicine.

In a more black and white world, doctors assumed that they had done the best thing for the patient. In our more modern probabilistic world we want to know if in reality we have favorably altered the course of events. Have we increased the sum of human happiness? When does the prevention, early diagnosis or treatment of one process permit the person to die of a more lingering and unpleasant process? If all women over the age of 50 follow the recommendations of the American Cancer Society for mammography, how much morbidity and mortality will occur during trips to the mammography unit?

For years, doctors reporting on the outcomes of specific treatments have excluded the persons treated who died from other diseases. This is not helpful to the person who wants to know what is going to happen to him. The disease excluded may be the one he would prefer to terminate his life.

Each of us practicing medicine knows that doctors caring for patients are concerned only with outcome in that person. The other 99 making up the probability table are of no immediate interest to them. If they believe there is a chance of a life-threatening disease whose hand may be stayed for a few months or years, they will cheerfully submit the 100 to great expense, discomfort, and some morbidity to identify the treatable patient. Indeed, when tens of thousands are considered they may even tolerate some mortality from the prescribed treatment.

Doctors in practice tied to individual patients will never willingly practice probabilistic medicine. Not knowing the dollar worth of a human life, expense will be no deterrent. Society may limit their life-saving focus but medicine will not.

There is more hope that doctors may become more aware of probabilities when they are faced with a diagnostic problem. Doctors, presented with patients with symptoms pointing toward the heart, take some history, perform some sort of physical examination, and usually order an electrocardiogram and x-ray of the chest. They have the option of ordering oblique films of the chest, films during inspiration and expiration, fluoroscopy of the heart, CAT scan, examination by ultrasound, or a variety of radionuclide studies. They may order an exercise test with EKG monitoring, exercise test using a variety of radionuclide imaging techniques, cardiac catheterizaton with visualization of the coronary arteries, coronary angiography with ergot derivatives to induce coronary spasm, determination of pressure gradients in coronary arteries, and a series of invasive procedures to test the responsiveness of the conduction system of the heart.

The tests that they elect to perform may be sequenced in a variety of ways. Doctors do not know the amount of new information that each test will yield. The information already obtained from history, physical examination, chest film, and electrocardiogram has caused the doctor to form a tentative plan. If the complaint is chest pain on exertion relieved by rest, with a normal-sized heart and a normal resting EKG, the doctor has a plan for caring for this class of patient. What are the tests which can so increase the specificity of the pathology that they will alter the plan devised in the absence of the test? In many instances the disease category—for example, coronary arterial disease—has already been established and more tests are ordered because the doctor is looking for information that bears on prognosis.

The collection of data on outcome and the sequencing of tests in different orders give the information needed by the bio-statistician to determine the probability that the test in question will alter the probability of disease or the probability of a given outcome sufficiently to alter the behavior of the doctor as he cares for the particular person in question. A study of this kind has recently been done by the group at Duke Medical Center who have evaluated the information added by an electrocardio-graph-monitored exercise test. They found that the exercise test added no measurable prognostic information after cardiac catheterization had been performed, and the information added before coronary angiography was quantitatively small and unlikely to change the behavior of the doctor.

This type of study offers a better chance of interesting the doctor in the probabilistic world than does the question of life or death. The system, even so, has in it a tremendous amount of inertia. The doctor likes to order tests, third party payers like to pay for tests, the health industry likes to sell the technologies, and hospitals like to capitalize and profit from the technologies. I can hear angry cries saying it's not so. I never listen: I just observe. Observation indicates that I am right.

Chapter 25 ⌒

Uniqueness of the Elderly Patient

E lderly persons who live independent lives compose a large part of the practice of family physicians and internists. These doctors know that the elderly are fragile and rebound more slowly from any type of injury. They know that inflammatory processes, be they pneumonia or appendicitis, cause a less violent reaction in the elderly than in younger persons. They know that drugs are metabolized more slowly and that iatrogenic diseases are easy to produce. They know but may forget that aging is a chronic process. The doctor must always keep in mind that his patient may outlive his financial resources. He needs to guard his patient's resources and be certain that only useful procedures are prescribed.

When elderly persons can no longer live independently the structure of the practice of their doctor may no longer meet the needs of the aging person. A variety of community services, including nursing, day care centers, physiotherapy, communication specialists, home maker, meals–on–wheels, occupational therapy, and personal knowledge of governmental agencies that can give financial aid are needed. Patients who are legally blind are eligible for special services. One needs to know ways to tap the services of groups offering support to patients with Alzheimer's disease, muscular dystrophy, multiple sclerosis, osteotomy problems, et cetera. At this level, geriatrics becomes a specialty separable from the care of independent persons.

Geriatricians have the responsibility to guide their patients from the time of loss of independence until death. They are the gatekeepers who make sure that no independence is lost that can be prevented by modern medicine, and they protect their patients from the young eager-beavers who try to achieve technological results that are not yet achievable. They work out plans to conserve the energies of family and friends and decide in advance how any life-threatening situations are to be handled. Competent geriatricians have most of their patients receive terminal care in their place of residence and few in an acute care hospital.

Dependent elderly patients require the services of generalists who are good diagnosticians and comfortable with information obtained from history, physical examination and a small number of laboratory tests. These patients have multiple disease processes, most of which are static. They have developed a philosophy of living and have many interesting and bizarre notions about health. They are looking for a friend they can talk with, and they do not require that their doctor cure them.

The elderly population has certain needs. They need to be listened to. Histories emerge slowly with many seeming irrelevancies. Interviews and examinations of elderly patients have to be paced. The entire picture emerges slowly and over time. The physical examination of the elderly patient does not always have to be complete. It has to be helpful. Careful evaluation of mental status is important in evaluating an elderly patient. Remember that unhappiness, depression, drugs, fatigue, poor hearing, and loss of vision may cloud the picture. Prudent use of biomedical technology is essential. Look for what can be helped—not what can be diagnosed. Help the family handle dementia and paranoia. A careful distinction between biologic depression that is drug-sensitive and unhappiness that is drug-insensitive must be made. An arm around the shoulder does more for unhappiness than all the drugs in existence. Finally, a plan for medical emergencies agreeable to the patient, the family, and various support organizations should be discussed early in the care of the elderly patient.

Geriatrics, more than any other area, highlights the differences between doctors who treat diseases that occur in people and doctors who care for people who have diseases.

IV

The Right to Live and the Right to Die

*T*he fun of medicine really lies in helping people to perform in a way that they wouldn't perform without you, to keep them alive when they wouldn't be alive without you. The terminal part of the world, namely, the business of helping a patient intelligently and painlessly get out of this world, is a necessary function of physicians, and they should be taught to handle this part of their practice. It is not where the gold lies, it is not the exciting thing about being a doctor, so while I have written about death and dying, I look on it as a part of being a professional, not what gives happiness to the day.

Chapter 26

The Setting of the Problem

*W*ith us always has been the question of when the life of the individual begins and when society begins to protect this life because it has gained the dignity of a human being. Eggs and sperm die separately without any pangs of conscience. "The pill," as commonly used, prevents ovulation and does not cause the death of the fertilized egg. When the egg and sperm unite, a process is initiated that will produce a highly individualized, unique person. "The pill" can be used in large doses to prevent implantation of the fertilized egg. What are the ethical and legal complications of this use of "the pill"?

The doctor has always accepted the responsibility that the survival of frank monsters is not in the best interests of society, and no unusual means are employed to keep them alive. Many mentally defective children have correctable associated defects. Correction of these defects, particularly when they involve the cardiovascular system, may prolong life for many years without modifying mental capacity. What frames of reference should the doctor use in determining in which of these children corrective surgery should be done?

Death was once an agreed-upon end point. This has ceased to be true. Every day, persons in whom the heart and respiration have stopped are restored to life and return to normal activity. On the other hand, we have patients who are still alive because respiration and circulation continue although the brain has ceased to function.

The medical profession is trained to save life. If a condemned criminal is hurt before the time of his execution, a team of doctors and nurses will work all night to keep him alive and to restore him to health. Doctors' instincts are to prolong life. They have seen many people die after prolonged efforts. They have seen great hardships result from keeping alive persons who can never again contribute to family life or to society. How do doctors and the patient families determine when doctors should become passive?

Depressed patients may commit suicide. If this can be prevented, most patients will recover. All doctors agree that prevention of suicide of a depressed patient is a responsibility of the medical profession. What legal and ethical considerations should guide the physician when a non-depressed patient attempts to take his own life because he faces dishonor or incurable illness?

Patients under Medicare are supported in our hospital only as long as they can be shown to continue to profit by the care. Most ill patients will live longer if they remain in the hospital than if they are sent to a nursing home. How do doctors determine at what point Medicare benefits stop? In past years these matters were usually determined administratively by the county commissioners. It was their responsibility to discontinue funds for hospitalization and they were not, usually, overly concerned that, without hospitalization, death would occur sooner. Now these decisions are being placed more and more often with the doctor. What legal and ethical considerations guide the hospital utilization committee in such decisions?

To what degree does the patient or the family control medical treatment and when does society make the decision which may disregard the wishes of the individual? Most will agree that adults who are rational can decide their own fate. The matter becomes more difficult when minors are involved. Shall a child in danger of dying from hemorrhage receive a transfusion if it is against the wishes of the family? Who should make the decision and on what grounds?

The successful development of care units for patients with myocardial infarction and the successful treatment of previously fatal kidney failure raise the most acute problems of living and dying.

Many patients are alive and active today because of the prompt use of external cardiac massage, electrical defibrillation and mouth-to-mouth breathing. There is suggestive evidence that coronary care units not only can restore the dead to life but, by careful monitoring and proper use of drugs, can prevent the change in cardiac rhythm that will cause death. These units are expensive. They create enormous demands for trained manpower. How much of the resources of the country should be devoted to the care of the population beyond the age of 40 who clearly have a limited life expectancy when compared to the neglected, preschool child of three?

The time of dying in patients with kidney failure is now largely an administrative matter. Renal dialysis and transplantation would allow additional years of life for many of our patients. Each such life prolonged for a year or more represents a large investment of money and manpower. The program raises many ethical considerations. Does every man so love his brother that he will give him one kidney? Kidneys of people who die can be used for transplantation if they are promptly harvested after death. This takes agreement and planning during the life of the donor. What protection does the donor have that his own life will not be shortened to benefit the recipient? Should the organs of a dead man belong to the family or to society?

The fun of medicine really lies in helping people to perform in a way that they wouldn't perform without you, to keep them alive, when they wouldn't be alive without you. The terminal part of the world, namely, the business of helping a patient intelligently and painlessly get out of this world, is a necessary function of the physician, and he should be taught to handle this part of his practice. It is not where the gold lies, it is not the exciting thing about being a doctor, so while I have written about death and dying, I look on it as a part of being a professional, not what gives happiness to the day.

Chapter 27 ⌒

Dependency

I t is easy to be a good citizen until one reaches the age where dependency overtakes us. We have not yet found an easy or graceful way for most of us to leave the stage on which we performed adequately as independent persons.

I know of no way to make dependency as attractive as independence. The devotion of all our resources to the care of the dependent elderly would not make old age as attractive as youth.

We have to face a most difficult issue: what level of care do we want to give to what groups of persons? Professionals in aging have rarely faced this problem directly. They want more of everything and would have the surroundings and personal services equal to those of the independent population.

We have accepted that comatose persons who have dead brains may be declared dead even though circulation and respiration can be maintained. Will we in time accept dementia as slow dying, and when it disconnects the patient from his surroundings, will we make no attempt to prolong life? In a demented person, what is the purpose of the medical procedures, the administration of food and water, the use of antibiotics, the daily vitamins, the polypharmacy? It is not to help the patient enjoy life. Too much of the brain is dead. We care for the partly dead person because we have not developed an ethical or religious system that allows us confortably to call it quits. We are afraid that we will become dehumanized if we don't postpone death. The care is for the living and not for the dying. We face the same issue with birth control and abortion. The egg, sperm, and embryo never complain. It is the feelings of the persons who live that are at stake.

When I have cockroaches in my living quarters, candy in every nook and corner, a refrigerator filled with rancid food, and have stopped bathing, I won't care. My children will be appalled and want to instigate change. They are afraid I'll break my hip and die before I'm found. If I'm institutionalized, what is the minimal acceptable care that society can offer me?

The same ethical considerations and the same feelings of frustration at having no workable ethical frame of reference confronts us as we care for patients with expensive medical technology who have only one chance in 100 of being restored to a life they can enjoy. In the old days it was simpler. In 1930 Dean Wilburt Davison,[1] a renowned pediatrician, came to the medically underserved Southeast. He was in great demand as a consultant who could work out a care plan for demented children who placed heavy demands on the family and community. The consultation had some aspects of a festive occasion. When Dean Davison got down to business, he requested everyone except members of the family to leave. He then determined who was going to contribute personal services or money for support of the child. He asked all other family members to leave. The final hard choices were then made by persons who had to implement them from their own resources.

In our day the family is not dependent on their own resources. They have a variety of community, state and federal resources to cushion them. Insurance coverage, Medicare, Med-

---

1. Wilburt C. Davison was the first Dean of Duke Medical School and Professor of Pediatrics, and established the first faculty of Duke University Medical Center.

icaid, state and community agencies dilute the feelings of personal responsibility. If we let patients finish the act of dying without intervention, we must ask ourselves: are we letting demented persons die because we don't want to pay more taxes? Are our actions moving us to tolerate a new holocaust because there is no ethical basis for non-intervention?

It is interesting that we have devised cultural and ethical systems that allow us to kill millions of healthy persons without feelings or guilt. We have a name for that system. We call it war. Until we have a philosophical and ethical system which accepts death as a part of life and acknowledges that the last part of living is the first phase of dying, we will make no progress. How will we develop an ethical base for new types of behavior? I assume that it will come about by forces tangential to problems we are discussing today.

Two changes in our culture have occurred by a tangential approach. Knowledge that cancer is caused by exposure of our bodies to a variety of chemicals has changed much of our behavior. You no longer have to put out ash trays when doctors congregate in large groups. Workers in chemical plants are forcing management to adopt new methods of reducing exposures. Years ago no one thought that prevention of cancer would be possible and that prevention would produce major changes in our lives. Cancer in many situations is now recognized as the work of man on biological systems. It is no longer an act of God.

Eventually a new generation will come to believe that there are limits to the amounts of money and services they are willing to expend for persons who have suffered "brain death" which prevents them from relating in any way to their environment. The concept of partial brain death and ways to deal with it will emerge. By one device or another, a system of behavior compatible with this belief will evolve, and society will permit the partially dead to complete the act of dying in peace.

Many families and doctors have allowed death to come quietly and painlessly to patients with terminal cancer. Patients permanently out of touch with their environment may be allowed to die from infections if they have expressed this desire in a living will, or if the family requests the withholding of anti-microbial drugs.

We need to take a new small step and define the boundaries of partial brain death which permits some demented persons to die as they would have died in the home many years ago. In those days food and drink were offered, but no actions were taken if the patient did not eat or drink.

It will take time and thought to define the syndrome of partial brain death which allows the withholding of antibiotics and feeding, by spoons, by tubes, and by intravenous fluids. There is no hurry; it took several years to define total brain death and to make organs available for transplantation from a person with a dead brain to a living recipient.

We do not want to move quickly or become involved in legal issues. We simply wish to define the state of partial brain death which allows families not to force food and drink on persons whose brains will never allow them to relate in any meaningful way to their environment. This is a small step, but one that would relieve the suffering of many families.

Meanwhile we struggle with the economics of home and institutional care. I've no objection because we must fill in time until forces that we have not yet anticipated mold our attitudes.

Chapter 28 ☞

The Need for a New Look at
Geriatric Care

A ll societies have had to solve the problems created because a minority of the people at any one time require personal services and material assistance beyond the amount that is needed by the majority of persons who are healthy and able to work. Babies, children, handicapped persons, and people who become dependent because of mental problems, unemployability, or advanced age have in common the need for support systems that are more extensive than those needed by healthy, adult working persons. The distinction between the dependent and independent portions of our society is clear-cut when one compares a productive machinist and a baby. The distinction becomes more hazy when one considers the support system needed by single working women with one or more children and the support systems needed by workers if occupational illnesses are to be prevented.

The older persons in our society present no special problems as long as they are financially solvent and can maintain the style of living that they maintained as productive members of the work force. As they lose their independence and become dependent upon other members of the society, they raise all the issues, ethical and economic, common to dependency. The geriatrician cannot through medical skills solve the problems of dependency but can bring to these issues a broad perspective colored by everyday experiences obtained by working with the elderly.

Progressive Increase in Number of Dependent Persons

In an earlier period, many persons believed that education and improved health care combined with advanced technology would reduce our dependent population to well babies, healthy children, and chronologically very old persons. They envisaged that support systems for sick and handicapped children and for persons with chronic illness, and welfare for adults unable to fit into the work force, for adults with mental disabilities, and for other disadvantaged groups would require less and less of our resources. Unfortunately, the complexity of our society has increased rather than decreased. In the years 1966 to 1976 the number of persons permanently limited in their activities because of health conditions increased by 37 percent with a much larger proportion of those disabled claiming to be unable to carry on their main activity. During this 10-year period, our population increased by only 10 percent.

Many persons who can function independently in a rural family-centered society lose their independence when they have to meet the much more complex demands of an urbanized society. Medical science and technology have increased the salvage rate of fetuses and have allowed the survival but not the restoration to independence of many damaged children, accident victims, and elderly persons. In most instances, the private and public sectors still behave as if the problems of dependency will go away, and planning is done on an *ad hoc*, fragmentary basis.

Societal Options

The number of dependent persons in our society is increasing more rapidly than the number of workers. Even if the present ratio of dependent persons to workers should remain unchanged, the dependent population would consist of many more of the elderly and fewer of the children. The demography of the work force also is changing. Welfare children of today and the children of black and Hispanic minorities will form an increasing percentage of the work force of tomorrow. In the future, we will be forced to make one or more of the following changes.

1. Increase taxation to the point where the United States becomes a completely socialistic society.
2. Develop programs in which partially dependent persons barter some services with other partially dependent groups.
3. Pay a minimum wage to every partially dependent person who can do some work. The source of the wage would be in two parts: Part A paid by the dependent person using the services, and Part B paid by public monies to bring the income of the employed person to the level of the minimum wage.
4. Establish a national service corps and require all persons capable of working to give their services to the country for a period of 2 years. Payment for these years would be at the subsistence level.
5. Allow persons who are demented or likely to die within a few months to die without the intervention of modern medicine and technologically oriented support systems.

I do not believe that taxation to the point of loss of most freedoms for everyone is desirable, and I will not comment further on this alternative.

Barter services have real possibilities. Many mothers barter baby-sitting services. In a community of older dependent persons, exchange of services which allows persons not to be institutionalized is common. Bartering can be done without additional funds.

Bartering breaks down when one person has become so dependent that he or she has no services to barter. It does not work well when the income of the person bartering the services is below the subsistence level. A combination of income support that would allow a dependent person with some financial resources to purchase services at a level below the minimum wage from another, less dependent person who was, in turn, supplemented by public monies to bring his or her income to the level of the minimum wage is a possible solution. The greatest obstacle to this solution is the rigidity of the federal and state bureaucracies. They have trouble in crosslinking two areas—welfare and support for the dependent—into a single system.

The establishment of a national service corps where every person gives two years of service to the country and fellow citizens without expecting to be rewarded materially is a possible solution. We have a demand for services which cannot be met by paying salaries at rates now set by the public and private sectors without increasing taxes to the point where we forgo our capitalistic society. Two years of services is a small price to pay for a lifetime of freedom. The material returns to the young people in the corps would be small; the rewards of unselfish service would be large.

The concept of service might well be extended beyond the two years required for the young before they would become permanent members of the work force. Each of us could well give one week of service per year during our entire working life.

Our society has not faced directly the issue of allowing designated groups of persons with dementia, or with a 97 percent incidence of death within 3 months, to die from the withdrawal of support systems. We have, of course, faced this issue indirectly. Many persons in our country, and literally millions of persons in undeveloped countries, die each day because of lack of food, shelter, sanitation, and medical supplies. We are not interested in paying taxes to prevent these deaths. Perusal of state psychiatric institutions, state homes for children who have to be institutionalized, prisons, blighted central cities, and pockets of rural poverty indicates what we are willing to pay for and shows that planning is done on a fragmentary, *ad hoc* basis.

Much money is spent on persons who will die or become demented within three months. As we improve our ability to define who will die or become demented within three months, we will be under increased pressure to conserve money and accept the inevitable. I for one would rather spend the money on increasing the opportunities for children with healthy bodies and brains.

We hesitate to do by direct planning what we do by passive neglect. The ethical issues involved are many and will be avoided by the healthy workers until the material costs of not facing the issues become too high. The emergence of birth control, of new sexual freedoms, of the independent childless woman, and of the number of married couples with none to two children shows that behavior can change. Society is not static.

The Physician-Geriatrician as an Expert Whom the Society Legitimately Expects to Exert a Leadership Role

The geriatrician caring for the dependent population must consider all the issues listed above and give intelligent leadership to the body politic in these areas. The issues are the tax monies for dependent persons, their distribution among the various dependent groups, and ways to give the agreed-upon quantity of services without destroying the freedoms of the rest of society.

Once we face up to how much comes the more difficult decision of to whom. What is due the low income, welfare, and minority mothers whose babies, if properly nourished and educated, will form a sizable portion of our work force? What is due the babies who appear normal? What is due the premature baby who can be kept alive by our support system whose death a few years ago would have been certain? What is due the premature baby who can now be kept alive but only at a great risk for permanent handicaps? What is due the deformed baby, the autistic child, the children with major brain defects, those with sickle cell anemia, and the endless list of conditions that result in dependency? How much is due the persons who are dependent because of social conditions—disabled veterans, accident victims, victims of criminal assault, drug addicts, tobacco-induced cancer patients, the people who populate our prisons, and alcoholics? How much for the population with no education who have lived by physical labor and who are unemployable at the age of 55? How much for the dependent elderly who can live at home with some support? How much for the demented elderly who recognize no one?

The answers to the above questions will reflect the beliefs of individual persons, of small and large groups, and of our society as a whole. There are those who believe the best answer is to provide maximum services and who are willing to borrow to pay for them with the assumption that our children and children's children will have new sources of wealth to pay back the borrowing. Others are more conservative and are more willing to set limits.

Setting limits on the dollar value of services to be supplied is difficult, but even more difficult is the decision as to the distribution of the services. Unwanted pregnancies of today produce persons who may be dependent for the next 60 to 100 years.

Welfare children of today are our potential workers for tomorrow and our potential future welfare clients. Some of our dependent persons have intact brains, some are totally demented, and a number are comatose.

When financial and family resources are available to the individual patient, responsible decisions on what services are meaningful and should be purchased can still be difficult. How should the time and resources of the family be distributed among a demented great grandmother, the incontinent and dependent grandmother, the working mother and father, and the children in the family? The decision is even more difficult when one must decide how much of public monies are to be spent for support of each member of the family when the mother and father are unemployed. Equal amounts of money and resources spent on each member of the family would not solve the problem. The cost of creating a personalized and clean environment for the demented great grandmother would exceed that needed to support the young, healthy child of an alcoholic mother.

Is every unborn fetus and every person with functioning respiration and circulation to have a support system establishing an environment which would be satisfactory to the person living independently in our society? As one would expect, each of us gives a different answer when we are personally involved. Then we want maximum support. The level of support provided to care for the severely deformed and mentally deficient children, for the mentally ill, for those on welfare, for those unemployed, for prisoners, for drug and alcohol addicts, for many disadvantaged minorities, and for the aged gives our collective answer. When we are not personally involved, we will settle for a very limited support system, and we will tolerate living conditions for dependent persons that are far below the standards achieved by the independent portion of our society.

The physician who becomes a geriatrician needs to see the

broad sweep of problems that face society as it cares for dependent elderly and uses up resources that could be available for education of children. When resources of a family are limited, how should they be distributed among three or four generations? Should the physician hold off and let pneumonia be the friend to ease the old person out of this world? If a fractured hip is repaired to relieve pain in a demented elderly person, should death from the operation be prevented by antibiotics and blood transfusion? Is it ethical for nondepressed persons facing inevitable deterioration of mental and physical facilities to arrange for their death by drugs?

While the generalization that dependency in old age presents the same problem as dependency at other times of life may be true, there is at least one tangible difference: in old age the inevitable outcome is death, and before death there will be a steady loss of function. The adult population can look at other causes of dependency and not identify with them. Old age is different. Every vigorous, active adult knows that he or she will have to die suddenly or join the dependent aged at some time. The fact of the matter is that age eventually distorts our bodies and minds and makes us unattractive. This projection into the future creates fear in many people who are not at peace with the biological facts of birth, reproduction, aging, and death. Combined with low pay scales, it results in a shortage of qualified persons to care for the dependent aged.

Role of the Physician-Geriatrician in the Care of the Elderly Person

The geriatrician can help in the transition from independent living to dependency and can frequently postpone the dependency by using every community resource to provide home care and transportation. For those who prize independence above all else, the geriatrician can persuade the family, friends, and social agencies to allow the older person to assume certain risks. Many elderly people are willing to assume the risk of a broken hip and an unattended death in order to remain independent. The old know that death is inevitable. It has happened to their friends.

The physician has the responsibility to be certain whether the cause of the dependency is remediable. He is a gatekeeper to prevent any dependency that can be reduced or removed by scientific medicine. In a low socioeconomic group with substandard medical care, the alert geriatrician will find a number of remediable medical problems. In a well-cared for group of elderly persons of higher socioeconomic status, the geriatrician will make few ten-strikes that will remove dependency.

In older persons who have decreased functional reserves in every system, acute illness can cause a rapid change in mental state, and the patient can no longer direct any aspect of care. The experienced geriatrician will have talked with the family and with the older person, and they will have agreed on a course of action to be taken when acute illness occurs. Many families do not want a cardiac pacemaker to be replaced if the patient is demented. They may not want the first pacemaker inserted in life-threatening situations if they know that the patient is existing rather than living. A decision as to whether antibiotics, intravenous fluids, blood transfusions, respirators, or cardiopulmonary resuscitation are to be used can usually be decided in advance of the acute problem. If the patient is admitted to a general hospital, care can be sharply directed to the acute problem, and the usual routine of the hospital can be broken.

It is not an easy matter to handle the feeling states created among the nursing and attendant staff when the end result is inevitably death and when the plan of care accepts death as a legitimate outcome. The amount of nursing time devoted to healing a small decubitus in a patient who is alert and responsive should be greater than the amount of nursing time spent on a large decubitus in a person so demented as to be unaware of the decubitus. The distribution of staff time is one of the areas where the geriatrician can be of real service to the nursing staff.

The family of a patient who is becoming senile and showing paranoid changes needs a great deal of help. They have to appreciate that the brain is failing and that the patient is unable to modify his or her behavior. The family knows intellectually that the behavior, including fecal and urinary incontinence, cannot be controlled by voluntary effort, but they have a hard time integrating their intellectual knowledge into their own feeling states. As mental deterioration starts, a cycle of multiple complaining frequently begins. The patient knows that he or she is not well, and bodily complaining is the only way to express this feeling. This type of complaining, if not understood, can cause the family and physician to keep searching for a definitive treatable cause. None is found, and the complaining is not modified by drugs. Acceptance and understanding by family, attendants, and physician are the only answer. An arm around the shoulder, a walk down the hall, a glass of warm fluid are helpful.

The family has the greatest trouble with paranoia directed toward themselves, and nurses and attendants also have trouble with paranoia directed toward themselves. Attendants who care for the elderly frequently come from the lowest-paid group of workers and are apt to belong to minorities whose feelings are easily bruised. Racial slurs by the paranoid elderly patient are not uncommon. The only solution is in an understanding of behavior when the structure of the brain is deteriorating. The physician is responsible for bringing this level of understanding to the family and attendants.

The loss of independence, the fact that one's financial resources are either depleted or being depleted, and the death of close friends and associates do produce unhappiness in many elderly persons. Many physicians do not differentiate clearly between unhappiness that is built into the situation and the disease called depression. In our experience, unhappiness is not drug-responsive. A human touch is the only alleviating therapy.

The question of suicide as an acceptable end for the elderly has yet to be faced by the medical profession and society. Traditionally, we are taught that taking one's own life is equivalent to the diagnosis of depression. I do not believe this is true. Knowing the inevitability of death, one may decide on an intellectual basis that elective death is better than slow degeneration. The problems of elective dying present many hazards, and they frighten us as individuals. We wish to make the election and not have it made for us. Nevertheless, this problem will not go away. In time, mechanisms will be developed to allow the nondepressed person to have a greater role in determining the time and method of dying.

I have presented the problems facing persons who cannot support and care for themselves without special help. As long as the brain functions, each dependent person may enjoy fruitful and rewarding days. The role of the geriatrician is to see that this possibility is translated into reality for elderly persons. When medical science has nothing further to offer, good care can ensure that each day is as pleasant as possible. Geriatricians want society to spend its money where the return is greatest. They recognize that eventually scientific medicine has only a relatively minor role, and they assume the more rewarding role of helping supply good social, economic, and cultural support systems.

Chapter 29

The Right to Live and the Right to Die

T o be alive, to grow, to achieve, to reproduce—these are the drives of the young. To enjoy, to reap the fruits of labor, to give a helping hand to others, to make a more useful society—these are pleasures of the middle-aged. To live in contentment until death draws the shade—this is the goal of the old. Many of the old know the difference between living and being alive. They want to live as long as they are thinking persons who can enjoy the day. They want the time between the beginning of death (senility) and the cessation of respiration and heart beat to be as short as possible.

In past generations, pneumonia or other bacterial infections were looked on as the old person's friend. Today these formerly fatal infections are controlled, and we have many more elderly persons who continue to live long after they have lost contact with their surroundings. These persons frequently are cared for in nursing homes where the family cannot have sustained contact with the administration of the nursing home and has little to say about the medical treatment of the aged relative. When the person in the nursing home develops new symptoms, he is frequently moved to a hospital where he receives intensive diagnostic and therapeutic services, directed towards preserving heart beat and respiration. The doctor, ignorant of the background of the patient, must try to preserve the heart beat and respiration.

After a few days or a few weeks, the patient is returned to the nursing home for continued existence. This sequence of events may be repeated several times before death finally occurs.

The cycle cannot be broken until our culture accepts dying as a part of the cycle of living and is willing to prepare for death as the final drama of life. Death in one's prime is a disaster; death as a final act terminating our normal lifespan is a blessing.

Many persons, including myself, have written out instructions for their personal physician so that he can be guided if they suffer brain damage or become senile. The doctor knows that the family accepts the fact that the nursing home, hospital or home can be used as a place to die with dignity. Intravenous feedings, stomach tubes, catheters, antibiotics, oxygen and tracheotomy are not needed. Comfort for the patient and minimal scars for the living who are left behind is the goal of the care.

Chapter 30　⌒

If I Become Ill and Unable to Manage My Own Affairs

T his is the first generation in which the majority of persons 40 to 60 years of age are financially responsible for three generations. Each family with children has at least four grandparents and, in this day and age, at least one of the grandparents will survive and become partially or completely senile. This last week, I have been shopping for a very sweet but beginning-to-be-confused grandmother.[1] She is used to doing for herself and she does not adapt easily to having other people do for her. She tells her house-helper not to do most things. She intends to do them herself. But, alas, she forgets and they are never done. She likes the visiting nurse who helps her with personal cleanliness and gives her advice about cooking, eating and shopping but, again, she cannot believe that she can't go it on her own.

As I shopped in the community where she has spent her life, I found good will on all sides. The saleswoman in the department store, the assistant manager of the bank, the salesman responsible for mattresses, pillows and linens were interested in my problem: how to keep my lady functioning and living in her community. Each of them has faced similar problems. They look on the nursing home as inevitable but each, on the basis of his

---

1. Harriett Selby, Evelyn Stead's mother, died at the age of 94 of a chronic illness.

own experience, hopes that time can be postponed. They have no good answers to old age—nor do I.

What shall we do if Grandmother slips and breaks her hip? What shall we do if she develops pneumonia? Must medical science intervene and keep her breathing but not living?

Our family must face the problem and advise Grandmother's doctor of our feelings. We, as parents, must remember that the patterns we devise for our parents are likely to be followed by our children when they must make similar decisions.

Many years ago, I wrote my own personal physician a letter to guide his hand if I became ill and my mind was not functioning normally. I quote from that letter:

"If I become ill and unable to manage my own affairs, I want you to be responsible for my care. To make matters as simple as possible, I will leave certain specific instructions with you.

"In event of unconsciousness from an automobile accident, I do not wish to remain in a hospital for longer than two weeks without full recovery of my mental faculties. While I realize that recovery might still be possible, the risk of living without recovery is still greater. At home, I want only one practical nurse. I do not wish to be tube-fed or given intravenous fluids at home.

"In the event of a subarachnoid hemorrhage, use your own judgment in the acute stage. If there is considerable brain damage, send me home with one practical nurse.

"If, in spite of the above care, I become mentally incapacitated and have remained in good physical condition, I do not want money spent on private care. I prefer to be institutionalized, preferably in a state hospital.

"If any other things happen, this will serve as a guide to my own thinking.

"Go ahead with an autopsy with as little worry to my wife as possible. The Department of Anatomy crematory seems a good final solution."

Now the time has come to write a letter to Grandmother's doctor. He is a wise man and will appreciate the support the family can give in a problem for which there is no wholly satisfactory answer.

V

To Young Colleagues

*H*ow can you achieve happiness in your life? There is no magic answer, but there are some general guidelines.

Chapter 31

A Talk with Young Colleagues about Their Future

I 've enjoyed my career, the fun of interacting with my attractive and perceptive wife, with three intelligent, achieving children and three even more attractive grandchildren, and with a host of intellectually brilliant colleagues. My support system has been so excellent that I've not felt very needed and I've never known whether I was really intellectually viable on my own. My colleagues have been hard on my ego but certainly essential to my accomplishments.

Many young doctors have come to me for advice about their professional careers. I have been impressed with the fact that they rarely ask what I think is the most important question: How can I achieve happiness in my life? There is no magic answer, but there are some general guidelines. I would like to share them with you.

Remember that each person is unique. Define the activities that give you the greatest satisfaction. All forms of work are equally honorable but not all create equal satisfactions for a particular person. Medicine is demanding. Most doctors who really enjoy their professional life make little distinction between work and play. Both require you to be awake and to score points. You will have the most fun when you have selected work games and play games at which you excel. The field of medicine is broad enough so that you can find your proper niche.

The years immediately after medical school are the freest you will ever have. Spend them in a way in which each year repays you in terms of satisfaction, achievement, and personal growth. Do not worry about whether each year represents progress towards some elusive career goal. Collect payment for each year in full as you go.

Select a mate who has joy in living and work towards the goal of romantic love. Mutual respect and admiration are the essential elements for a longtime relationship. Fun in bed can usually be achieved if the couple means for the marriage to succeed and if the bonds of respect are high. When a couple marries, the idea of true romantic love is an illusion. The notion that you have found the only one in the world who can give you joy cannot be defended. After 40 years of successful marriage, when each member of the pair has been slowly molded to fit the other, romantic love becomes a possibility. Evelyn and I are now molded by each other to the point where no other persons can equally well fit our individual needs and personalities. We are now uniquely suited to each other and romantic love is a reality.

Children can add to the joy of the day. Don't have them until you are willing to give something of yourself each day to them. Keep the accounts current, and close the books each day at midnight. You have had your fun and they owe you nothing.

Don't become a complete materialist. There are other satisfactions than things. Always live below your income. Have the bills paid before Santa Claus comes.

Arrange your free time in a way so that all the family can enjoy each other. Building a house together has given parents and children in our family a common interest and mutual respect. I am pleased that, in spite of my having lived a full and busy professional life, none of my children has felt neglected by their father. When your children grow up, respect their individuality, accept their differences, and do not require them to be like yourself or like each other.

Become a student of human behavior. Learn that behavior is determined by the structure of each individual brain. Some elements of the brain are reversible but most are not. Knowing that brains limit behavior leads to true tolerance of one's fellowman. Establish high requirements for those born with the most flexible brains. Do not make sadistic demands on those who cannot achieve the highest levels of performance. Appreciate the fact that selection is more important than education. Arrange to accentuate the best qualities of those you have selected and minimize their weaknesses.

Accept the reality that happiness is finite rather than infinite. When happiness has reached a reasonable level, stop and enjoy it. If you make the error of thinking that happiness is infinite, you will chase "the little man who is not there" and miss the enjoyment of the present. This knowledge can allow you to beat the Peter Principle and prevent you from being promoted to your level of incompetence.

Your life is your own. Live it.

Sources of Eugene A. Stead, Jr., Essays

Page 1.   This passage was an introduction to "A Way of Learning" and was originally published in Continuing Medical
Education Newsletter, X, no.9, September, 1981. It was sub-
sequently edited for "A Way of Thinking" by EAS in February, 1995.

Page 3.   Stead, E.A., in Hippocrates Revisited. R.J. Bulger,
Editor, Med Com Press, 1973, N.Y., pp. 126–129; *What
This Patient Needs Is a Doctor,* edited by G. Wagner, B. Cebe,
and M. Rozear, Carolina Academic Press, Durham, NC
1978, (WTPNAD), pp. 135–138.

Page 7.   Continuing Medical Education Newsletter X, no. 9,
September, 1981.

Page 13.   E.A. Stead, Jr., Happy, Communicative and Understanding Doctors—The Roles of the "Humanities" and Bioscience, *North Carolina Medical Journal,* 47:561–562, 1986.

Page 19.   E.A. Stead, Jr., Thinking Ward Rounds, *Medical
Times,* 95:706–708, 1967; WTPNAD, pp. 25–27.

Page 23.   E.A. Stead, Jr., Preparation for Practice. *The Pharos*
29:70–71, July, 1966; WTPNAD, p. 21.

Pages 27, 31, 37.   E.A. Stead, Jr., Where One Stands Determines What One Sees. *The Pharos* 45:27–32, 1982.

Page 43.   E.A. Stead, Jr., Physicians: Past and Future, *Archives Int. Medicine*, 127:703–707, 1971; WTPNAD, p. 61.

Page 55.   WTPNAD, p. 168.

Page 57.   *J. Clin. Invest.* 32:548–549, 1953. Presented as the Presidential Address at the American Society For Clinical Investigation. Atlantic City, N.J., May 4, 1953; WTPNAD, pp. 147-152.

Page 63.   E.A. Stead, Jr., Soma Weiss: The Characteristics that Made Us Know He Was a Great Man, *The Pharos* 50:11–12, 1987.

Page 69.   E.A. Stead, Jr., Jack Myers and Medicine, a talk given in honor of Jack Myers on the occasion of his retirement from the University of Pittsburgh in 1983.

Page 75.   The Thorndike Unit at Boston City Hospital: 1937–1939, by E.A. Stead, Jr., in "The Harvard Medical Unit at Boston City Hospital" vol. II, part I: The Peabody Minot Tradition, 1915–1950. Commonwealth Fund Publication, The University of Virginia Press for the Frances A. Countway Library of Medicine, Harvard Medical School, Boston, MA, 1983, pp. 332–337.

Page 89.   E.A. Stead, Jr., "Just Say For Me," F. Schoonmaker, E. Metz, Editors, World Press, Inc. Denver CO, 1968; WTPNAD, p. 13.

Page 91.   E.A. Stead, Jr., Good Will Toward Men, *Medical Times*, 94:1535–1537, 1966; WTPNAD pp. 73–76.

Page 93.   WTPNAD, 69–73.

Page 99.   E.A. Stead, Jr., Brain Sorting, *Readings and Perspectives in Medicine*, Booklet 8, Medical History Program, The Trent Collection and Irwin A. Brody Fund, Duke University Medical Center, Durham, NC 1983.

Page 117.   E.A. Stead, Jr., Health and Illness, *Medical Times,* 96:753–754, 1968, WTPNAD, p. 81.

Page 119.   E.A. Stead, Jr., Traps and Stratagems of Diagnosis, *Medical Times.* 95:588–589, 1967; WTPNAD, pp. 15–16.

Page 121.   Interviews of BFH with EAS May 16, 1991 and February 24, 1995.

Page 123.   E.A. Stead, Jr., The White Bear Syndrome, *Medical Times.* 97:256, 1969.

Page 125.   E.A. Stead, Jr., The Use of the Fundus to Demonstrate the Complexity of Communications. *North Carolina Medical Journal.* 44:617, 1983.

Page 127.   E.A. Stead, Jr., Two Lessons. *North Carolina Medical Journal.* 51:7–8, 1990.

Page 131.   E.A. Stead, Jr., Patients That Recover. *Medical Times.* 95:802–804; WTPNAD pp. 57:59.

Page 135.   "Our Probabilistic World" is an unpublished essay written in May, 1982 from a discussion of EAS with Frank Starmer, Ph.D., a faculty member in computer science and statistics at Duke University.

Page 139.   The essay "Uniqueness of the Elderly Patient" was presented as a lecture to the Tennessee Valley Medical Assembly on October 1, 1984.

Page 143.   From an interview of EAS with BFH on March 4, 1992.

Page 145.   E.A. Stead, Jr., The Setting of the Problem. *Medical Times,* 95:1173–1175, 1967; interview of BFH with EAS, March 4, 1992.

Page 149.   Unpublished essay on "Dependency" presented as a lecture at Conference on Geriatrics, Houston, Texas organized by Kathleen G. Andreoli, March 25, 1985.

Page 153.   E.A. Stead, Jr., The Balance Between Freedom, Public and Private Enterprise, and National Service: The Need for a New Look at Geriatric Care. *J. Amer. Geriatric Soc. USA*, pp. 30-33, 1982.

Page 165.   From an unpublished National Academy of Medicine, Institute of Medicine, Report of a Meeting on "Death and Dignity" by E.A. Stead, Jr., June 10, 1971.

Page 167.   E.A. Stead, Jr., If I Become Ill and Unable to Manage My Own Affairs, *Medical Times*, 98:191–192, 1970; WTPNAD, pp. 173–175.

Pages 171, 173.   E.A. Stead, Jr., from a speech given to the Association of American Physicians on the occasion of EAS acceptance of the George M. Kober medal in May, 1980; *Trans. Assoc. Amer. Phys.* XCIII:38–39, 1980.

Sources of Illustrations

Frontispiece, Back Cover. Eugene A. Stead, Jr. Photograph by Ronald L. Usery in 1992 (used with permisson of the North Carolina Medical Journal).

Endcover. Barton F. Haynes. Photograph by Lewis Parrish.

Page 79. James E. Paullin. Photograph courtesy of Duke Medical Center archives.

Page 80. Soma Weiss. Photograph courtesy of Duke Medical Center archives.

Page 81. Henry Christian. Photograph courtesy of Duke Medical Center archives.

Page 81. George Minot, William Castle, Soma Weiss. Photograph courtesy of Duke Medical Center archives.

Page 82. Eugene A. Stead, Jr. Photograph courtesy of Duke Medical Center archives.

Page 83. Resident Staff of Grady Hospital in 1946. Photograph courtesy of Duke Medical Center archives.

Page 84. The Department of Medicine at the Peter Bent Brigham Hospital, 1941. Photograph courtesy of Duke Medical Center archives.

Page 85.   Eugene A. Stead, Jr. teaching Duke Medicine House-staff. Photograph courtesy Duke University Department of Medicine archives.

Page 86.   The House that the Stead Family Built. Photograph by Barton F. Haynes in 1995.

Page 87.   Eugene A. Stead, Jr., age 86. Photograph by Barton F. Haynes in 1995.